BrainTap Technologies

Disclaimer: This book is designed to provide information in regard to the subject matter covered. It is sold with the understanding that the publisher and author are not engaged in rendering psychological advice and the processes in this book are non-diagnostic and non-psychological. If psychological or other expert assistance is required, the services of a licensed professional should be sought. The purpose of this book is to educate and entertain. Neither BrainTap Technologies, the author, or any dealer or distributor shall be liable to the purchaser or any other person or entity with respect to any liability, loss, or damage caused or alleged to be caused directly or indirectly by this catalog or the contents made available in it.

Copyright ©1995 – Updated 2017 by Patrick Kelly Porter, Ph.D. All rights reserved, Without Prejudice U.C.C. 1-207. No part of this publication may be reproduced or transmitted in any form or by any means, electronic or mechanical, including photocopy, recording or any information storage system now known or to be invented without permission in writing from Dr. Patrick Porter except by a reviewer who wishes to quote brief passages in connection with a review written for inclusion in a magazine, newspaper, video or broadcast. Violation is a federal crime, punishable by fine and/or imprisonment. Title 17, U.S.C. Section 104.

ISBN: 978-1-937111-08-3
Printed in the United States of America

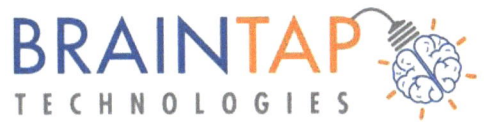

Table of Contents

Featured Programs 5

BrainTap Headset 7

Abuse
- Healing Meditations for Child Abuse Survivors 9

Addiction
- Freedom from Addiction Series 10

Alcohol
- Alcohol Series 11

AM
- AM Series 12

Autism
- Children's Opportunity for Brilliance 12

Brain
- Alpha, Delta, and Theta Training 13
- Brain Fitness Breakthrough 14

Cancer
- Coping with Cancer 15
- Say No to Cancer 16

Childbirth
- Stress-Free Childbirth 17

Children's
- Optimizing Your Children's Inner Potential 18
- Enlightened Children's 19
- Consciousness - Children's 20

Christian
- Christ-Centered Energy Meditations 21
- Gospel Meditation 21
- Christian Weight Loss 21

Dentistry
- Stress-Free Dentistry 22

Diabetes
- Diabetes 22

Fasting for Health
- Fasting for Health 23

Gluten Free Lifestyle
- Gluten Free Lifestyle 23

Grief
- 8 Steps to Coping with Grief 24

Health
- Vibrant Health 25
- **Article:** 5 Simple Steps to Optimal Health 26

Heart Health
- Heart Healthy Lifestyle 27

Irritable Bowel Syndrome
- Freedom from Irritable Bowel Syndrome 28

Learning
- Accelerated Learning System 29

Life Improvement
- Better Life Me 30
- Finding Love and Building Winning Relationships 30
- ICan 31
- Life Mastery 32

Lyme Relief
- Lyme Relief 33

Medical
- Medical Recovery Series 34
- **Article:** Meditation Switches Off Disease-Causing Genes 35

Meditation
- Connect Up Meditation 36
- Chakra Meditations 36
- Energy Center Meditation 37
- Journey of the Soul 37
- Journey to Egypt 38
- Meditation Basics for the Inner and Outer You 38
- Meditation Journeys 40
- Power Meditation 41
- Wandering Ninja 41

Menopause
- Mind Over Menopause 42

Musical Journeys
- Alexander of Sedona 43
- BrainTap Meditation Music 44
- Dominus Cervix 44
- Kinetic Harmonies 44
- Stargate Octium 45

Nutrition Series
- Nutrition Support 45
- Why Your Brain is the Best Pharmacy 47

Pain
- Knee Pain Relief 48
- Pain Free Lifestyle 48

Phobias
- Phobia Relief 49

PM
- PM Series 50

PTSD
- PTSD 50
- BrainTap Breakthrough for Military PTSD 51

Public Speaking
- Public Speaking Series 52

Sales Mastery
- Sales Mastery Series 53

Sleep
- Healthy Sleep Habits 54

Smoking Cessation
- Smoking Cessation Series 55

- **Article:** The Secret to a Perfect Night's Sleep! 55

Sports
- Blue Chip Mind of Championship Basketball 56
- **Article:** BrainTap Your Way to the Top of Your Sport 57
- Equestrian 58
- Mental Coaching for Golf 58
- Mental Edge Golf 59
- SportZone Series 60

Stress
- Stress Reduction 61

Wealth
- Abundance for Women 62
- Busting Loose from the Money Game 62
- Wealth Consciousness Series 62

Weight Loss
- Blissful Body Meditation 63
- Habits of Naturally Thin People 64
- HS Weight Loss 67
- Lipo-Light Ultimate Body Contouring Program 68
- Weight Loss Through Consciousness 68

Writing
- Screenwriting Visualization 69

Research 70

Featured Audios

How Can We Help You Change Your Life?

BrainTap's featured audios help restore your brain's natural balance, so you can operate at peak performance and acquire the positive new habits and lifestyle you want—naturally. Simply choose the custom-crafted, proven program that best fits your needs, or ask your health provider for guidance.

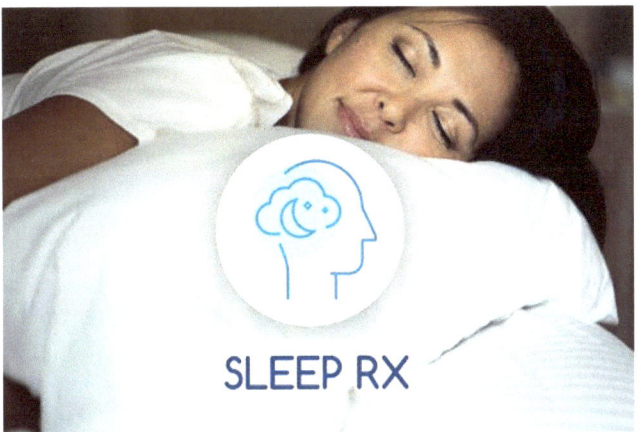

Do you suffer from unhealthy sleeping habits?

Did you know that not getting enough deep, restful sleep can lead to serious health issues? Our Sleep RX program was specially designed to help you easily and gently restore your body's natural ability to fall asleep. By retraining your brain and body to relax, your brain will begin creating proper sleep inducing patterns that will get you into a deeper relaxed state, allowing you to wake up refreshed and rejuvenated.

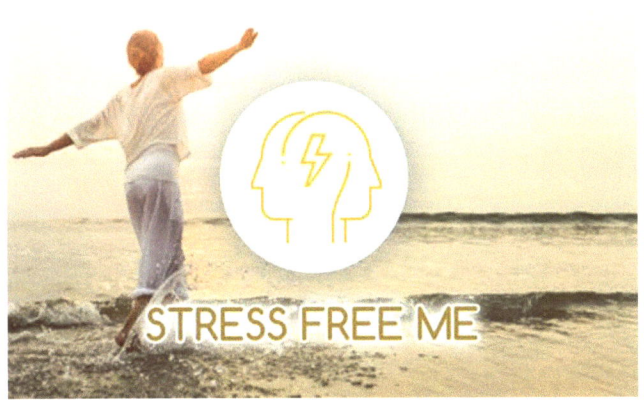

Is chronic stress robbing you of a great quality of life?

High stress keeps your body in constant flight-or-fight mode, causing an overproduction of stress-related chemicals, which can lead to significant health issues. Our Stress-Free Me program retrains your brain and your body how to react properly to stress, decreasing the chemical imbalance, keeping you more relaxed, and ultimately helping you stay healthier.

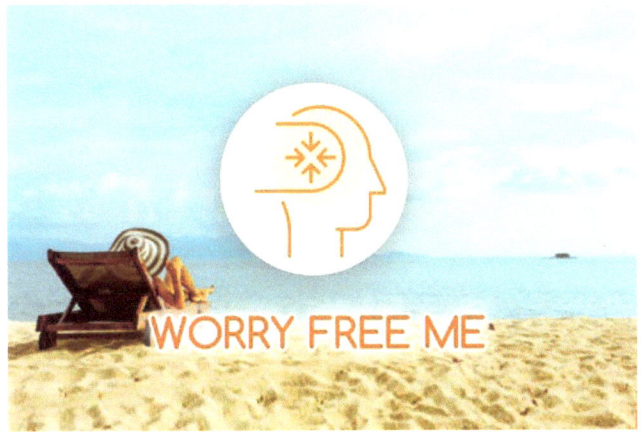

Are worry and anxiety overwhelming you?

Our Worry-Free Me program will ease the worry that's consuming your life by retraining your brain to relax, eliminating negative thinking, and ultimately giving you the ability to think through anxious feelings and situations rather than simply reacting to them.

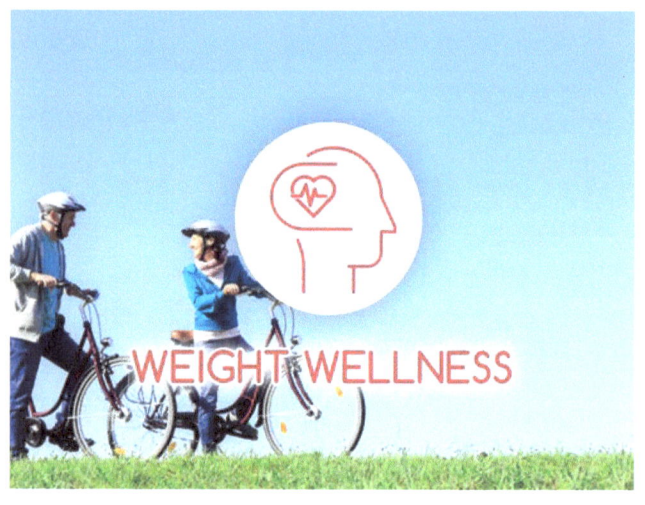

What do you do when diet and exercise alone don't work?

People say that proper diet and exercise are the keys to achieving a healthy weight. However, one very important element is missing from this equation. Our Weight Wellness program is specially designed to help you visualize your end goal, and achieve it! By changing how you think about a healthy lifestyle on a subconscious level, you can once-and-for-all correct eating habits and behaviors, have the true desire to exercise, and maintain your results with proper nutrition.

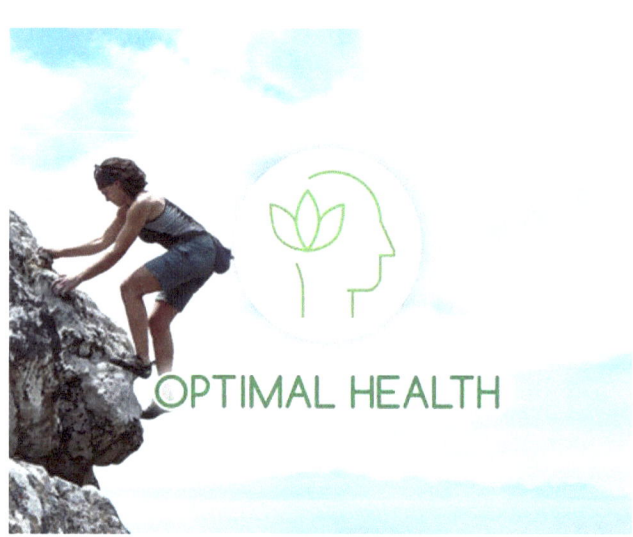

Do you struggle with maintaining balance in your life?

The meaning of *health* encompasses so many different elements from physical and mental, all the way to emotional, and most health-related goals are easy to achieve, but hard to maintain. Our Optimal Health program features sessions from various series that, combined, will help reduce stress and toxins, help you sleep deep and awaken recharged, boost your energy naturally, become more motivated, and help you develop healthy nutritional habits, so you will be able to achieve Optimal Health for life.

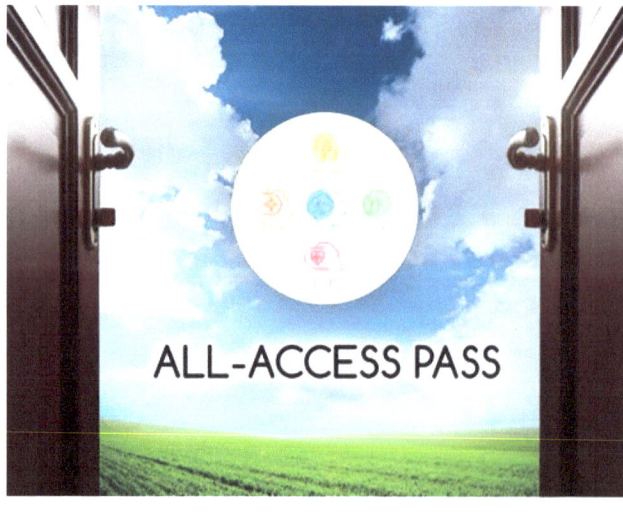

Looking for more ways to achieve the life you've always dreamed of?

It's easy when you have over 700 guided meditation audio-sessions available at your fingertips from our BrainTap mobile app. Choose from over 50 categories including: sports, pregnancy, menopause, cancer, PTSD, meditation, vibrant health, and so many more. We even have sessions designed especially for children! With our **All-Access Pass**, you and family can have it all!

Ask your health provider for more information about our **Featured Programs** or **All-Access Pass** and all that you can achieve in only 20-minutes a day with BrainTap! Or, visit braintaptech.com to find a provider near you.

Relax, Reboot, and Strengthen Your Busy Brain with the BrainTap Headset

Thousands of Men and Women Now Live Rich and Rewarding Lives Who Never Thought They Could...

Now you can see and feel the life-changing results that thousands of Dr. Patrick Porter's clinical clients have seen over the last three decades. These users report that regular braintapping with the BrainTap headset...

- Provided profound relaxation
- Fostered healthy sleep
- Awakened more energy
- Reduced brain fog and negative thinking
- Eliminated unwanted habits and behaviors
- Increased memory and focus
- Created peak performance!

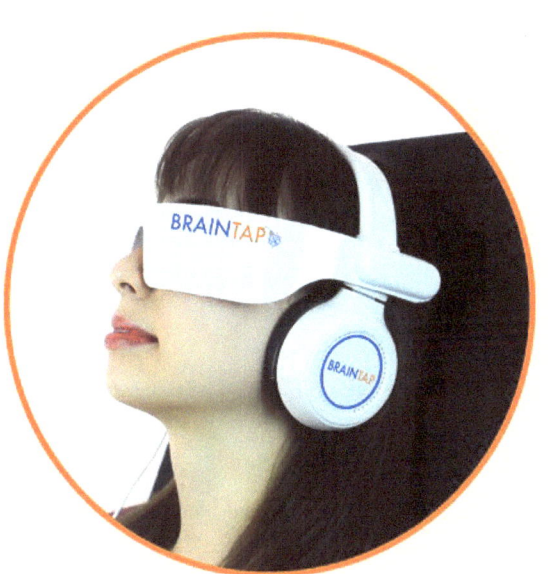

Whether you want to overcome stress eating or conquer a bad habit, instill a positive mindset, advance your career, master your sport, enhance your learning, get your body super fit, or simply regain the health you deserve, the BrainTap headset creates the enhanced brain states that will get you there faster and with less effort.

Experience the restorative power of LIGHT

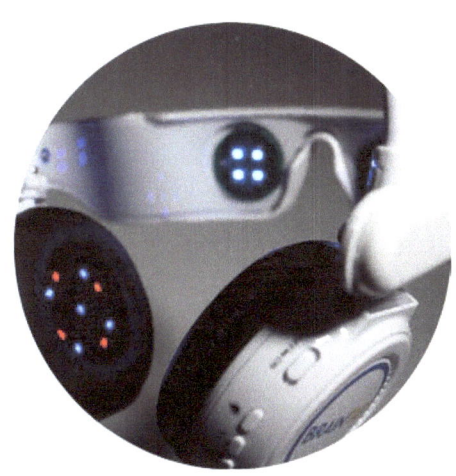

While the audios in the BrainTap Library feature powerful harmonizing tones, the headset adds a whole new dimension with the power of *light frequency therapy!*

Gentle light pulses delivered through the headset's visor send direct signals to the brain and **guide you into a deep relaxation.**

This innovative form of brainwave training is called *frequency following response*, and it provides <u>maximum results</u> in the <u>least amount of time.</u>

You simply slip on the BrainTap headset, start the BrainTap audio, lower the visor, close your eyes, and relax. You'll enjoy a braintapping session that is strategically encoded to take you way beyond what any power nap alone ever could!

But Wait...There's More!

In addition to the visual light show, the BrainTap also features **Auriculotherapy** – the delivery of light in the ears that activate trigger points, or meridians, and are known to directly affect the body's organs and systems. Activating these meridians is typically done using needles, but the BrainTap headset uses 9 LED lights, 5 blue and 4 red, in the earphones of the headset to achieve sublime serenity and balance...all without needles!

Let's put it this way...with the BrainTap headset, you don't have to spend 10 or 20 years struggling to learn meditation...but you can enjoy all the same benefits AND MORE in just 20 relaxing minutes a day!

The science says it all, but just look at what this expert has to say...

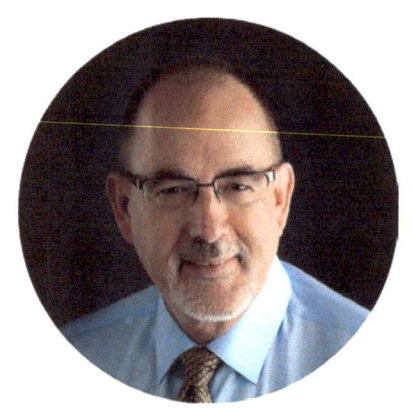

The BrainTap headset offers an advanced program in brain retraining, and I am pleased to endorse this product. We have been able to test the real-time brain response changes via the NeuroInfiniti EEG and demonstrate that it works as promoted. Nice work, Dr. Porter!

Richard Barwell, DC.
Founder Neurologically Based Chiropractic (NBC)
Developer of the NeuroInfiniti EEG

So, if you are the type who likes to get things done, here is your answer. Combining full-spectrum brain wave activity, left brain and right brain balance, enhanced circadian rhythm balance, natural energy, and a positive mindset to accomplish any goal you set for yourself, the BrainTap headset can help you achieve it all and more in only a few minutes a day.

The quality of Your Life is Directly Related to the Fitness of Your Brain!

Today, people spend thousands enhancing their bodies, but do nothing to improve the quality of their thoughts. The truth is, we can accomplish far more by managing brainwave activity and mentally rehearsing the positive, productive, and healthy lifestyle we all want. And with the BrainTap headset, it couldn't be easier!

Ask Your Health Provider for a complimentary demonstration of the BrainTap headset today -- or visit braintaptech.com to find a location near you.

Abuse

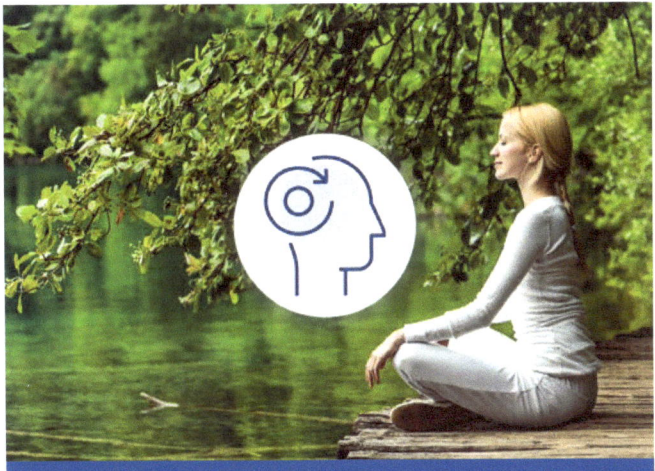

Healing Meditations for Child Abuse Survivors
Inspired by the Reaching Out Child Abuse Monument

This series by Patrick K Porter, PhD is inspired by Dr. Michael Irving's *Reaching Out Child Abuse Monument.* These sessions will assist you in seeing yourself as a remarkable person who has the courage to live through adversity, rising above and beyond a kind of cruelty that never should have happened. You will see that you have a hopeful, problem-solving spirit with a commitment to make more of your life. These meditations will help you recognize that the trauma occurred a long time ago. You now have the comfort of distance and the power to move forward. Listening will help you get grounded as you come to understand that a memory is not abuse; memories are thoughts and feelings, and are within your power to change.

IMPORTANT! This series is intended to address habits and lifestyle choices while enhancing spiritual faith and should never be used in place of professional medical or mental health intervention.

HMS01 – Meditation on Hope and Healing
You will let hope radiate through your spirit and will focus on thoughts that comfort, calm and heal. You will meditate on the people you can lean on for support and turn to for nurturing.

HMS02 – Meditation for Empowerment
You will meditate on feelings associated with your important accomplishments and how others see your strengths. You will come to trust your inner voice and intuition.

HMS03 – Meditation for Safety and Containment
You will explore what you need for your individual *safe room* and create it as your perfect place of relaxation. You will celebrate the power of resiliency and tap your inner wisdom.

HMS04 – Meditation for Healing Shame
Abuse survivors often carry a heavy burden of shame and humiliation. Here you will internalize the truth that the abuse was not your fault and that the shame does not belong to you.

HMS05 – Meditation on Trust
Abuse robs the birthright of trust. You will reawaken your innate ability to trust. You will explore what you need in your life and environment to feel safe and secure.

HMS06 – Meditation on Self-Soothing
You will nourish the positive and comforting feelings already inside of you. You will practice breathing in calming energy and releasing stress as you become more relaxed and self-aware.

HMS07 – Meditation for Grief and Letting Go
This meditation will support you in moving beyond the grief associated with child abuse. You will acknowledge the presence of grief and then give it permission to be resolved and released.

HMS08 Meditation for Healing the Inner Child
You will connect with the innocence of your inner child and help it make sense of the hurt from long ago, restoring your feelings of worthiness and reclaiming your ability to love and be loved.

HMS09 – Meditation on Celebrating Victory
You will focus on celebrating the victory of having survived and thrived through the adversities of childhood. You will reflect on the many ways you can be proud of yourself.

HMS10 – Meditation to Heal Self-Blame
Let go of the self-blame and the guilt and destructive behaviors that can accompany a history of child abuse. As you release self-blame you will feel joy and see yourself as a new you.

HMS11 – Meditation on Embracing Freedom
You will embrace and celebrate the freedom of having overcome the pain that lasted so long. This meditation will have you creating an ever-present force of freedom inside of you.

HMS12 – Meditation for Feeling Loved
You will reawaken the right to feel loved that was wounded by child abuse. You will reflect on times where you felt loved and notice where *being loved* exists inside you, so you can let that feeling grow.

HMS13 – Safe Mountain Meadow Retreat
You will create a safe mountain meadow retreat as an empowering inner sanctuary you can return to again and again. You will connect with the courage, bravery, and life skills you have inside.

Addiction

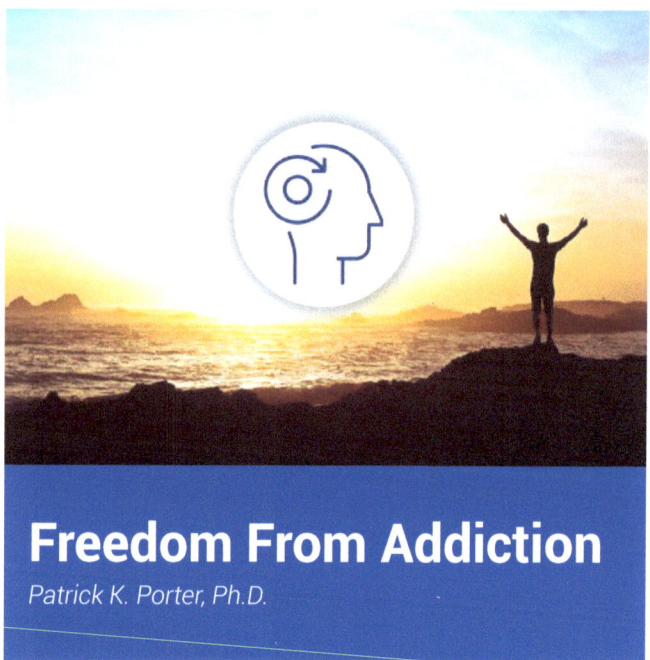

Freedom From Addiction
Patrick K. Porter, Ph.D.

Addiction comes in many forms, but the underlying cause remains the same. Every addiction has an underlying positive intention the mind is trying to fulfill. Now you can use the power of your mind to find more appropriate ways to satisfy that positive intention without the destructive behaviors of the past. This groundbreaking series offers new hope for a healthy new lifestyle to those suffering from just about any addiction.

IMPORTANT! This series is intended to address habits and lifestyle choices while enhancing spiritual faith and should never be used in place of professional medical or mental health intervention.

FA01 – Personal Responsibility and Working with Your Other-Than-Conscious Mind to Manage Your Life
Most people who struggle with addiction have lost their power of choice, but now you will rebuild your confidence and make new choices that will lead you to living an addiction-free life.

FA02 – Tapping into a Power Greater Than You to Restore Sanity to Your Life
Upon a simple cornerstone of faith, a spiritual structure of strength and resolve can be built. You will use your own concept of this higher power to start living the life you were born to live.

FA03 - Release Your Past and Embrace the Power of Change
You will mentally decide to turn your will and your future over to the care of the creator. You will relax and bear witness to the flow of life, and tap into its power, love, and grace.

FA04 – Taking a Fearless Moral Inventory
Even negative behaviors have a positive underlying intent. You will discover your positive intention and experience a mental cleansing and the release that comes when you forgive yourself.

FA05 – Developing the Courage to Express and Release the Past
Gain the courage to express your regret to those you have wronged in the past. Even though this is perhaps the most difficult step, it is also the most liberating.

FA06 – Discovering the Positive Intent Behind Old Behaviors
It is human nature to stay attached to old habits even when those habits no longer work. You will develop more appropriate habits, and you will come out the other side with positive new insights.

FA07 – Humility, Your Key to Lasting Change
Humility embodies the miracle of transformation, and all it takes is turning over the old unhealthy thinking patterns to your higher power.

FA08 - Trying New Things for a New Beginning
The key to lasting change is in having options. You will develop new ways of thinking and acting and life skills you didn't even know you had.

FA09 - Social Housecleaning from the Inside Out
You will clean up the bruised relationships and the pockets of guilt, pain, fear, resentment, and sadness inside you. You will release past hurts that may be stopping you from loving yourself and others.

FA10 - Becoming a Bridge-Builder for More Positive Relationships
Being a bridge-builder means that cleaning up your past becomes a way of life. You will learn to be vigilant over the part of you that wants to hold on to selfishness, dishonesty, resentment, and fear.

FA11 - Let Go and Go with the Flow (safe place)
You will create an internal compass to help you stay the course free from addiction. You will learn to keep your options in a safe place by keeping conscious contact with that power greater than you.

FA12 - Taking Care of Today by Planning a Bright Future
Learn to stay focused on the most important moment in time, which is now. By staying with a one-day-at-a-time philosophy, you can look forward to a bright and compelling future.

FA13 - Staying Connected to Your Higher Power
The secret to remaining free from addiction for a lifetime involves a spiritual awakening. Problem solving takes on a new level of creativity when you are connected to this power greater than you.

Alcohol

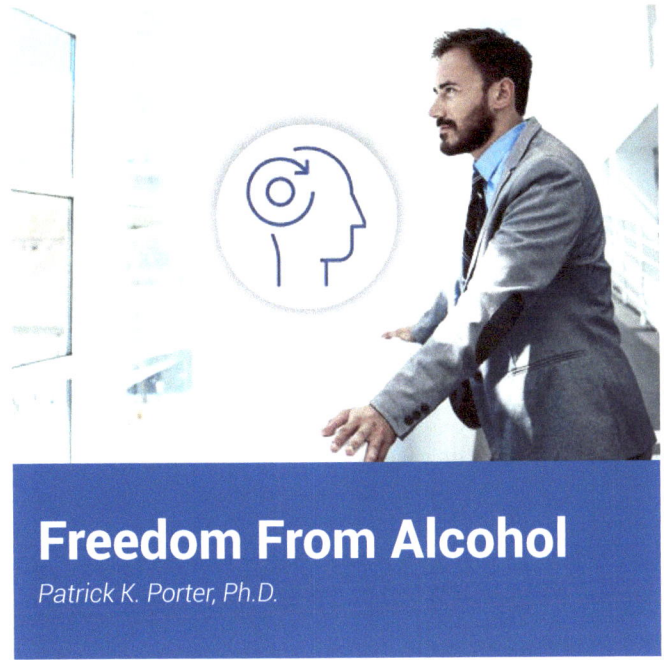

Freedom From Alcohol
Patrick K. Porter, Ph.D.

Patrick K Porter, PhD is the creator of **Hidden Solutions**, a program offered by the Arizona Health Council to help DUI offenders reclaim their lives. Now you can learn the hidden solutions that reside within you. You'll learn to form more positive habits and a healthy, balanced lifestyle. All you'll need to do is relax with these processes, which are based on Dr. Porter's personal experiences with his own addictive family and the twelve-step method that helped them heal. You'll quickly discover that the life you desire is within reach—once you tune into the unlimited power that is far greater than your conscious mind.

IMPORTANT! This series is intended to address habits and lifestyle choices while enhancing spiritual faith and should never be used in place of professional medical or mental health intervention.

AF01 - Breaking Beliefs and Behavioral Patterns
Alcohol addiction is often at the core of many emotional and relationship problems. Now you will view the problem from the creative right side of your brain where new options can be realized.

AF02 - Reclaiming Your Power
The first step to success is to admit that you are powerless over alcohol. Now it's time to retrain your brain by building your plan and then planning to succeed.

AF03 – Moving from Fear into Freedom
As you learn to trust in your guiding force, you will release the fear and frustration of the past and take back your power to create a healthy alcohol-free lifestyle.

AF04 – Using the Power of Intention for a Healthy Life
Engage your other-than-conscious mind to step into the alcohol-free life you were born to live. You will discover ways to de-stress, re-focus, and enjoy life more fully each day, one day at a time.

AF05 - Tuning into the Power of Change
Since the brain doesn't know the difference between real or imagined, you can comfortably admit to the exact nature of your wrongs so you can be free from the guilt of past behaviors.

AF06 – Gaining Freedom from Alcohol Step by Step
It's time to eliminate any negative thinking that may be keeping you tied to the debilitating effects of alcohol. Learn to forgive, forget, and move on with this unique healing process.

AF07 - Living Life Alcohol Free
Imagine the freedom you will experience by conquering the alcoholic behaviors of the past. Mentally rehearse living the rest of your life in health, wealth, and vitality with this calming session.

AF08 - Rebuilding Your Life
You will use this session to commit to leading an alcohol-free life in a way that's good for you and your family. How wonderful for you to now walk tall and proud without alcohol as a crutch!

AF09 – Taking Responsibility
You will visualize all people you have harmed and make amends. You will do this first in your mind and then, if appropriate, in the physical world.

AF10- Eliminating Negative Self-Talk
Now you can rid yourself of harmful behaviors and step into the alcohol-free life you were born to live. Learn to enjoy life more fully each day while you leave the shame and guilt in the past.

AF11 - Clean and Healthy and Loving It!
Once you've made it this far, imagine how great you will feel about yourself. This is a time for celebrating the brand-new mindset you've created.

AF12 – Mind & Body Solutions Alcohol Free
As you work to create the mind-body connection, a deep inner knowing of your true self will develop, keeping you focused on the best outcomes for you, your body, and everyone concerned.

AF13 – Awakening to a New Reality
Now that you have had an awakening, you will develop a lifelong desire to practice these principles in all your affairs, making the possibilities for your life virtually limitless!

AM

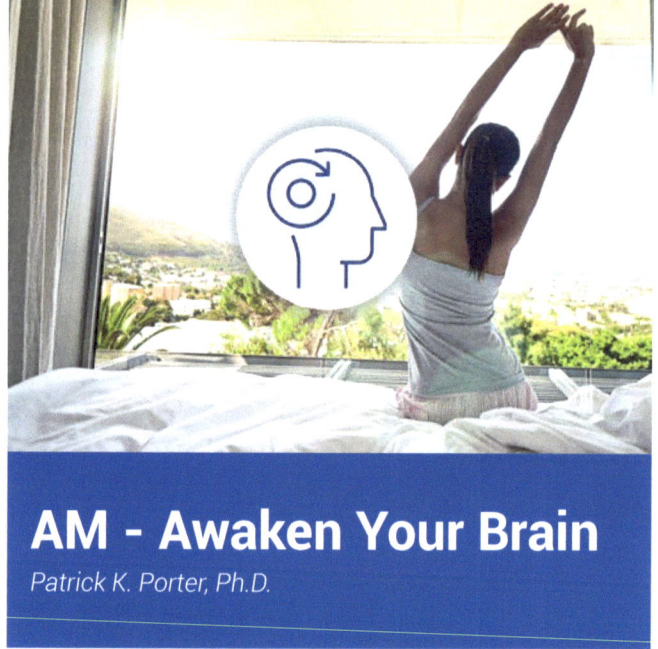

AM - Awaken Your Brain
Patrick K. Porter, Ph.D.

AM01 - Concentration
In ten easy minutes, you will visualize achieving your daily goals, boost your self-esteem, and at the same time enjoy greater focus and concentration.

AM02 - Focus
These ten short minutes puts you in the proper mindset to easily deal with distractions while staying on course to achieve your objectives for the day.

AM03 - Motivation
You will change procrastination into the confidence you desire. This session will help you become successful as you enjoy greater focus and concentration.

AM04 - Eliminate Negative Thinking and Start Your Day Right
Starting off the day with negative thoughts can automatically ruin your day. In this session, you will eliminate these thoughts and learn to excel throughout your day.

AM05 - Being Consistent with Exercise
Remaining consistent with exercise can be hard to do. During this session, you will focus on the word *consistency*, and learn the tools necessary to regularly exercise.

AM06 - Tap Into Infinite Energy
During this session, you will realize that thoughts turn into things. You will learn to tap into infinite energy and realize that it can be yours.

AM07 - Success One Step at a Time
Success as a whole may seem difficult to accomplish. In this session, you will find it easier to accomplish your goals when you take one step at a time.

Autism

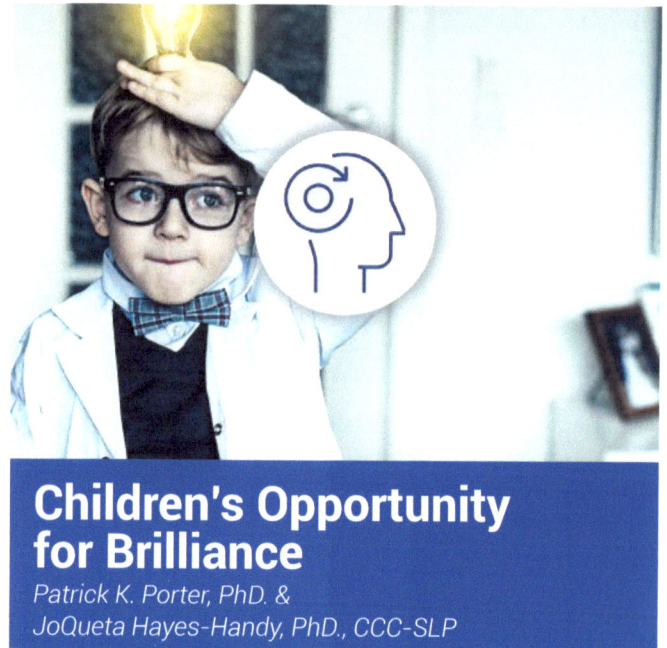

Children's Opportunity for Brilliance
Patrick K. Porter, PhD. &
JoQueta Hayes-Handy, PhD., CCC-SLP

JoQueta Hayes-Handy PhD, CCC-SLP, President, Children's Opportunity for Brilliance, a Nonprofit Organization, has teamed up with Patrick K. Porter, Ph.D. developer of BrainTap, to help create a breakthrough in learning for autistic children. The series combines the COB learning system with the brain science. Using the mind tools of rhythm, movement, and visualization, each session engages the student to exercise the brain and balance the nervous system. The results are a relaxed and more focused mental environment optimized for learning. The series is designed to build new neural pathways so the information gets linked to your child's prior knowledge for faster learning and better retention.

IMPORTANT! This series is intended to address successful learning habits and should never be used in place of professional medical or mental health intervention.

COB01 - Playing the Memory Game
With these lighthearted stories, your child will discover creative ways to recall auditory information for overall memory improvement.

COB02 - Tuning Your Brain, Hearing Your World... Auditory Processing
Your child will be building the ability to sustain auditory attention, along with the ability to better discriminate the sounds they hear.

COB03 - Adjusting Your Mind Lens, Seeing Your World
During this brain game, your child will experience accelerated visual processing exercises. Letter and number recognition and your child's fine motor skills will improve.

COB04 – Making the Connection, Processing Your World
The goal of this session is to improve overall processing speed. You will see improvement in working memory and interaction with peers.

COB05 – Tuning Out Negative Thoughts and Trying New Things
Autistic children commonly have intrusive thoughts (obsessions) that compel them to perform ritualistic routines (compulsions). Your child will break this pattern by creating comfort in change.

COB06 – Playing the Theater Game
Whether the goal is reading, adding numbers or expressing ideas with the written word, playing the theater game will help build focus in and out of the classroom.

COB07 – Playing the Relationship Game
This session is to help your child set goals and complete tasks by rehearsing using executive functioning. Your child will learn to think about one activity and then shift to another activity.

COB08 – Playing the Focus Game in Education
Whether the goal is reading fluency and comprehension, computation, or written expression, your child will mentally rehearse these steps until they become natural in everyday activities.

COB09 – Playing the Language Game Using Your Whole Brain
When children know where their bodies are in space and time, they can better go with the emotional flow. You will notice heightened self-esteem as negative associations around learning melt away.

> *Limitation is when you allow your future to be created out of your past.*
>
> ~Patrick K Porter PhD

Brain

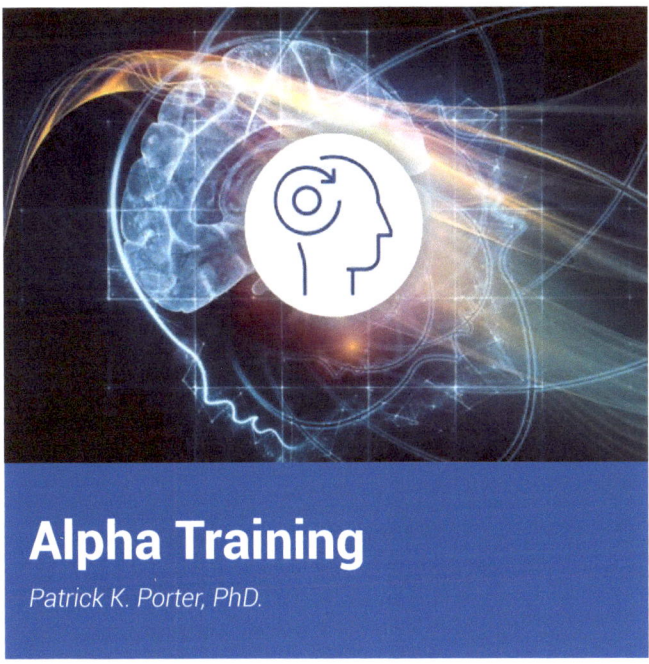

Alpha Training
Patrick K. Porter, PhD.

The alpha brainwave frequency is most associated with creativity, imagination, and flow. Alpha is the intuitive mind. It is also the brain state associated with relaxation, tranquility, and daydreaming. Flow thinking, or a state of *inward awareness*, takes place in alpha. It is also known as a super-learning state.

P08 – Quick Pick Up
In this session, you will listen to the beat and tones to increase your alpha brain wave activity.

P09 – Morning Boost
In this session, you will listen to the beats and tones that will give your alpha brainwaves a morning boost.

P18-P23 Alpha Training I-VI
In these sessions, you will experience a gradual increase of the binaural beats and isochronic tones to receive the maximum benefits associated with the alpha brainwave frequency.

Delta Training
Patrick K. Porter, PhD.

The delta brainwave frequency is deep, dreamless sleep. Delta is the unconscious mind. The BrainTap headset is designed to keep you from falling into this state of sleep, which is why the light and sound patterns change throughout the sessions. However, because these sessions stimulate a sleep cycle, nearly everyone experiences enhanced and more beneficial sleep.

P32-P34 Deep Delta Training I-III
In these sessions, you will experience a gradual increase of the binaural beats and isochronic tones to receive the maximum benefits associated with the delta brainwave frequency.

Theta Training
Patrick K. Porter, PhD.

This is the breakthrough state where you can reinvent your life. Theta is the inventive mind. It borders on sleep and is a meditative state with access to the other-than-conscious mind where you have higher levels of creativity, learning, and inspiration. It is also the state that helps you visualize and realize your goals.

15-30 MT With and Without Music
You will experience a gradual increase of the binaural beats and isochronic tones, along with music. This will allow you to receive the maximum benefits associated with the theta brainwave frequency.

P10 - Stress Magic
This meditative session will allow you to relieve stress while bordering between sleep and a meditative state.

P11 - Ocean Regenerate
You will relax and listen to the sound of the ocean in this session, while renewing your mind.

P12 - Bubbling Brook Relax
In this session, you will relax and enjoy the sounds of a bubbling brook.

P13 - Jungle Waterfall
You will listen to the sound of the jungle waterfall, which will lead to more beneficial sleep at night.

P14 - Forest Wind Chimes Balance
The forest wind chimes you hear in this session will bring balance to your mind and body.

P15 - California Coastline Dream
As you listen to this session you will hear the soothing sounds of the waves along the California coastline, moving you to a dreamy, drowsy state of relaxation.

P16 - Quiet Rain Drift Away
The sound of the quiet rain in this session will allow you to drift away into a deep, meditative state.

P17 - Hastens MindSpa Spring Afternoon
During this session you will listen to calming music, reminding you of a lovely spring afternoon.

P24 - Marrakesh
In this session you will travel to the city of Marrakesh, located in Morocco. You will drift into a meditative state while listening to the comforting sounds and visualizing this beautiful city.

P27-31 Deep Theta Training I-VI
In these sessions you will experience a gradual increase of the binaural beats and isochronic tones, in order to receive the maximum benefits associated with this deep theta brainwave training.

Brain

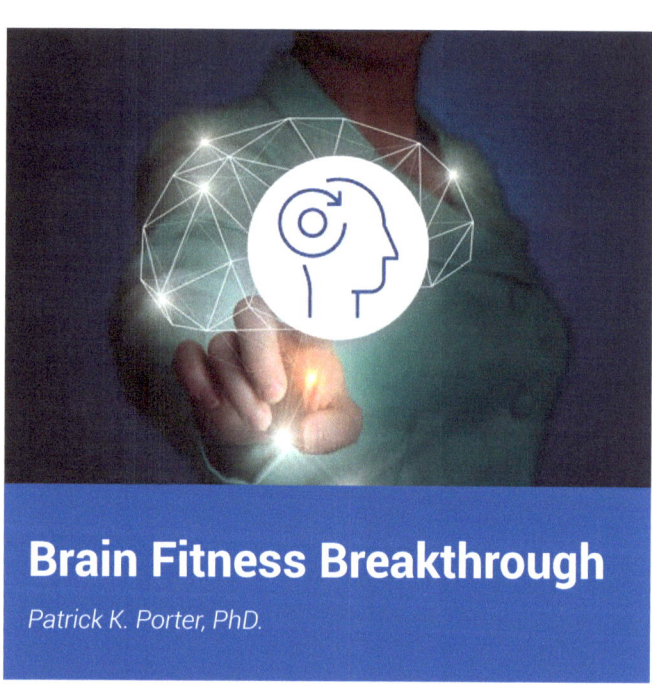

Brain Fitness Breakthrough
Patrick K. Porter, PhD.

Can you build a stronger brain? Research is now verifying that regular brain stimulation, and keeping the brain active, helps to improve and prolong healthy brain performance. These sessions are designed to train the brain to stay in a state of infinite possibility, and eliminate the old stuck states by using the science of Neuro-Linguistic Programming (NLP). The variety, diversity, and complexity of stimulation that your brain receives can make a significant difference regarding its performance. With these sessions, you can have some control over what stimulates and shapes your brain. Brain fitness is now as easy as kicking back and taking a quick nap.

BF01 - Being Fully Present - Increase Your Attention Span
In today's high-tech world, it's all too easy to lose focus on what's most important. These mental exercises will have you thinking more clearly and accessing skills that will improve your everyday life.

BF02 - Lightning Fast Problem Solving
Stressful situations can cloud your thinking. This thought experiment has been used by geniuses in the past to quickly master new skills and accelerate the learning of new information.

BF03 - Enhance Memory & Recall
Keep a keen memory of facts and look forward to using your life experiences for problem solving for the rest of your life.

BF04 - Creativity Booster
Life is about choices and effective decision-making, which is difficult without flexibility in your thinking. This session will boost alpha through a thought experiment to supercharge your imagination.

BF05 - Optimizing Your Brain's Capacity
As you stimulate creativity, focus, and concentration, you will find the things that you have done well in the past are improving, and those mental skills that need improvement are sharpening.

BF06 - Maintaining Focus & Concentration
You will build optimism about your brain's capacity to stay sharp. Being more alert is a natural part of maintaining a young brain.

BF07 - Achieving Peak Performance
We all experience moments of peak performance. You will capture that magical feeling, and recall those mental states of clarity whenever needed.

> *You are far greater than you've been led to believe and far more capable than you've yet allowed yourself to be.*
>
> ~Patrick K Porter PhD

Cancer

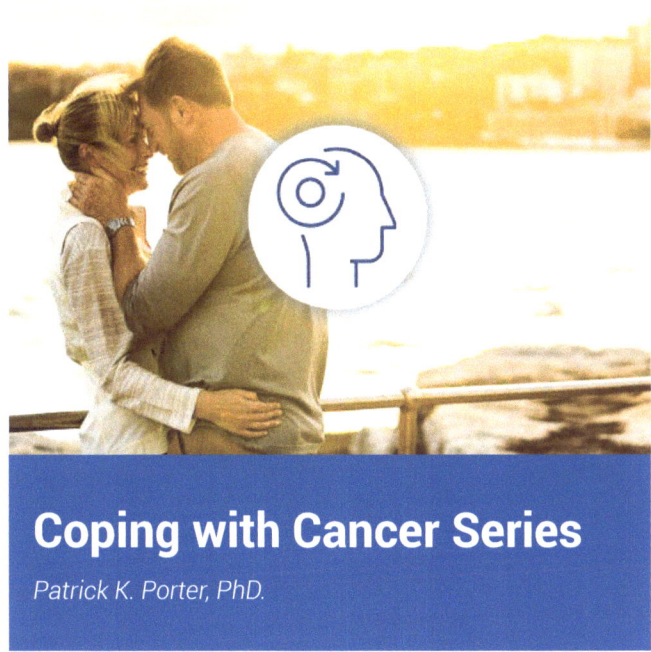

Coping with Cancer Series
Patrick K. Porter, PhD.

Being diagnosed with cancer is a stressful event—so stressful it can suppress your immune system and worsen the side-effects of treatment. Fortunately, through guided relaxation, you can let go of your fear and anxiety, and take charge of your recovery. Creative visualization can help you regain an optimistic attitude, spark your immune system, and maximize your medical treatment. If you are ready to join the ranks of people who have discovered the mind/body connection and its healing potential, than the Coping with Cancer series is for you!

IMPORTANT! This series is intended to address habits and lifestyle choices while enhancing spiritual faith and should never be used in place of professional medical or mental health intervention.

CWC01 - Relaxation for Inner Healing
In this first session, you will clear your mind of all negative or fear-based thoughts concerning your condition. At the same time, you will learn to allow the natural healing power of your body to take over.

CWC02 - Rejuvenate Your Body Through Deep Delta Sleep
You will release any anger or fear that may be interrupting your sleep while learning a simple method for returning to sleep if you awaken during the night so you can get the rejuvenating sleep your body needs.

CWC03 – The Power of Optimistic Planning
You will learn to inspire the positive emotions that create an optimum healing environment. You will awaken to the healing benefits of thinking positively even in negative situations.

CWC04 – Eliminate Harmful Habits for Health and Wellness
Perhaps a part of you wants to get well, while another part wants to deny the disease or is resisting giving up harmful habits. Now you can gain new life skills that will give you the best possible chance for beating cancer.

CWC05 – Tapping into Your Internal Pharmacy
Negative emotions such as fear, frustration, and anger can limit your ability to relax and heal. Now you can use your internal pharmacy to go with the flow, relax, and set a course for healing and wellbeing.

CWC06 – Focus on Health & Maximize Your Support Network
You will imagine your body absorbing the prayers and well wishes from friends and loved ones. You will be encouraged to do what you can to aid your recovery, such as taking walks or attending yoga classes.

CWC07 - Transform Negative Thinking into Positive Motivation
You will put external worries, such as money and housework, into proper perspective. You will learn about thoughts that harm and thoughts that heal, so you can focus your mind on the healing thoughts.

CWC08 – Build Your Own Internal Support System
You will learn to use your mind, the most powerful computer on earth, to regain your equanimity. Your mind has the capacity for virtually limitless problem solving and for helping you recover your emotional wellbeing.

CWC09 – Turn on the Power of Faith through Imagery
You will call upon a higher intelligence to help stimulate the white marker cells to do what they do best, seek out and destroy foreign agents in the body.

CWC10 - Using Goal Programming & Positive Expectancy
You will make your health your top priority. Setting healthy goals such as exercising, eating properly, and getting sufficient rest will keep you on the path to recovery.

CWC11 – Making Health a Priority and Staying Focused on Wellness
Build a positive attitude, gain the motivation to consume healing foods, to exercise regularly, and to feel that you are in harmony with your treatments. Uncover your deepest desires and values.

CWC12 – Supercharge Your Immune System
You will discover why thoughts are more powerful than things because thoughts create things—and the thing you will be thinking about is radiant health!

CWC13 – Relax & Let It Be
It is human nature to try to control everything—from family to friends to the health care system. This is the type of stress your body doesn't need. Here you will learn the secret to forgiveness and grace.

Cancer

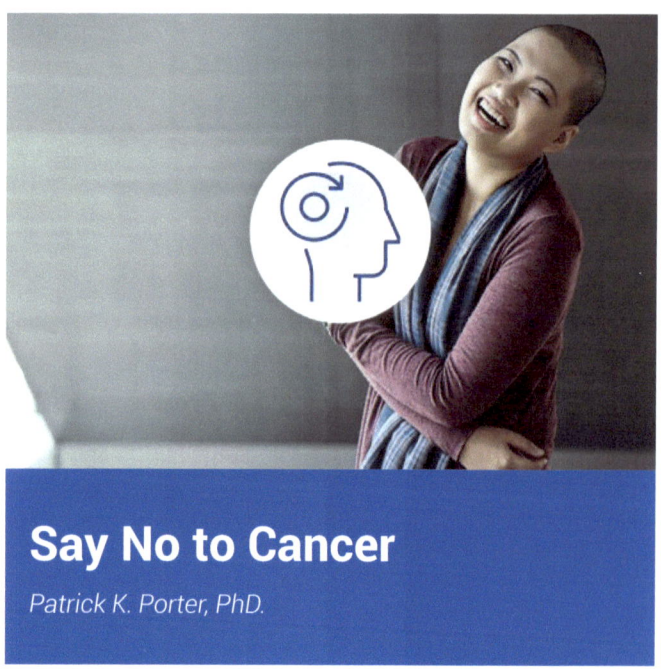

Say No to Cancer
Patrick K. Porter, PhD.

This series is based on the work of Carolyn Hansen's, Say No to Cancer. It has been proven that one of the main ways to protect your body against cancer is to avoid stress. You will learn to do just that when listening to these meditations. You will listen to your body, and recognize when you are responding to stress in order to minimize these emotional responses that many times are unwarranted.

IMPORTANT! This series is intended to address habits and lifestyle choices while enhancing spiritual faith and should never be used in place of professional medical or mental health intervention.

SNC01 - Eliminate the Fear of Cancer
The diagnosis of cancer is scary, however, you will learn to eliminate the fear of cancer and face it head on.

SNC02 - Take Back Control of Your Health
You have cancer, cancer does not have you. You will learn to regain control of your health with this meditation.

SNC03 - Living a Cancer-Free Lifestyle
You will transform your thinking and realize it doesn't take luck to avoid cancer. You will perform activities suggested in order to live a cancer-free lifestyle.

SNC04 - Quick Tips to Boost Your Immune System
You will use an NLP technique to learn important recommendations to put your health in high priority.

SNC05 - Healthy Mind - Healthy Body
You will transform your thoughts to focus on positivity. Once your mind is healthy, your body will follow.

SNC06 - Mind Trips for Dealing with Stress
In this meditation, you will concentrate on focus. Your body and mind will transform stress to relaxation.

SNC07 - Eating to Cancer-Proof Your Body
You will learn a technique called anchoring, which will train you to automatically think of certain feelings associated with eating healthy foods to cancer-proof your body.

SNC08 - Activate Your Strategy For A Long Disease Free Life
You will permanently change how you think of yourself. You will build a strategy and plan to succeed for a disease-free life.

SNC09 - Balancing Your Health Bank Account
You will recognize the benefits of using your health bank accounts and learn the importance of balancing your health deposits and health withdrawals.

Childbirth

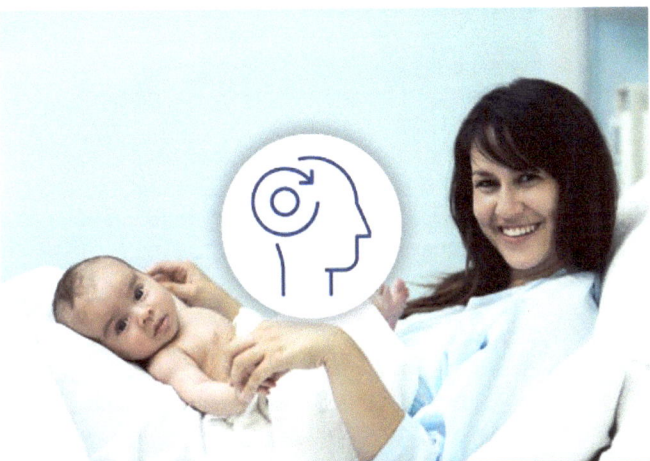

Stress-Free Childbirth
Patrick K. Porter, PhD.

Bringing a child into the world should be an amazing life experience. Sadly, for many women, the joy of the event is lost due to fear, stress, and pain. Also, research has shown that a fetus can feel the worry and negative emotions of the mother during pregnancy. Fortunately, with the discovery of the mind/body connection, women have an alternative. This breakthrough series is designed to help the mother-to-be relax, let go of stress, and enjoy the entire process of pregnancy, delivery, and motherhood. In addition, the listener is taught to use the power of thought to create an anaesthetized feeling that can transform pain into pressure throughout labor and delivery—making the entire process stress-free for the entire family.

CB01 - Visualize and Realize Your Pregnancy Goals
You will start experiencing the relaxation response, set healthy priorities, and prepare your body for the many changes it will go through for the next nine months and beyond.

CB02 - Mental Skills for Pregnancy and Delivery
Fear is a common emotion associated with pregnancy. You will gain the relaxed mindset and inner confidence you need for successful motherhood.

CB03 - Stress-Free Pregnancy by Design
When you are stressed, your baby feels it. Learn healthy ways to manage the stress of pregnancy. You will start using your mindpower to create a healthy environment for you and your newborn.

CB04 - Healthy Baby/Stress-Free Lifestyle
This session starts your training in creating that anesthetized state whenever and wherever you need it, along with the concentration and focus needed for a natural stress-free delivery.

CB05 - Emotional Readiness Mental Toughness
Being mentally and emotionally unprepared for delivery only adds to pre-existing stress. This session will build the mental toughness to convert fear into relaxation, allowing you to focus on wellbeing.

CB06 - Balancing Your Life During Pregnancy
During pregnancy you still have bills, housekeeping, and errands. You will gain an inner serenity as you build new life skills just as surely as you are building a new life inside of you.

CB07 - Building Flexibility Even When Frustrated
You will master open and clear communication so that your entire family can be a part of your pregnancy, and you will focus on your health and the health of your baby.

CB08 – Building Your Delivery Team
Your mind is your best labor coach. You will know how to ask your family or delivery team for encouragement and support. You will master a breathing and relaxation technique to combat discomfort.

CB09 – Going with the Flow...Transforming Contractions To Pressure
Mentally prepare for when your contractions reach peak intensity so that, with the power of your mind, you can feel only pressure, and keep your body as stress-free as possible.

CB10 – Quick Tricks for Stress-Free Delivery
By using this session, you will be ready to manage every aspect of your delivery. You will discover the keys to using your mind to accomplish your goals for motherhood.

CB11 – Preparing for Motherhood
You will be mentally, physically, and emotionally prepared for motherhood, so that even with a brand new person demanding nearly all your attention, you can regain balance in your life.

CB12 – Enjoying Life after Pregnancy
Learn to control the mood swings, anxiety, guilt, and persistent sadness that sometimes appear after childbirth. You will mentally rehearse your new lifestyle with joy and happiness for the entire family.

CB13 – Weight Loss and the New Mother
Once the new bundle has arrived and time commitments have changed, it's easy for a new mom to make her needs secondary. You make your health a priority and be able to lose all the weight you want, naturally and healthfully.

Children's

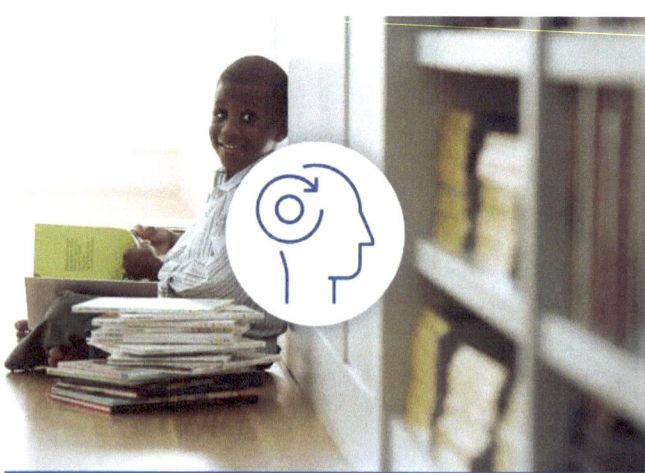

Optimizing Your Child's Inner Potential
Patrick K. Porter, PhD., &
Dr. Jared A. Leon, DC, CCEP, FICPA

Dr. Leon, with his specialty in neurology and physiology, and after using the BrainTap headset with patients and family members, saw a need for BrainTap sessions for the pre-teen to young adult age group. He approached Dr. Patrick K. Porter, Ph.D. with his innovative concepts for promoting healthy childhood development and a collaboration was born. This series consists of nine sessions, each one focusing on a different life skill today's children will need to succeed and flourish in the fast-paced, rapidly-evolving 21st Century. This series bridges the gap between the *Enlightened Children's Series* for small children and the *Accelerated Learning* series for adults.

OYC01 - Mastering Homework with a Positive Mood
Children learn correct breathing and the proper mindset for getting homework to the finish line. They remember to start with an end in mind.

OYC02 – Planning Happy Days at School
This session places special focus on being a great listener with all teachers. Children learn to properly sort memories, stay positive with friends, and create great memories for their future.

OYC03 - Mastering Confidence to Amplify Your Day
Confidence starts with the inner knowledge that you are loved. Your child will explore self-love and begin to own it. They will awaken the motivation to be a great starter and finisher of projects.

OYC04 - Having Fun and Laughing Often
As children practice building the skill of smiling and laughing often, they discover that laughter makes them feel great, that healthy laughter creates happiness and is one element to having fun daily.

OYC05 - Making Friends Easily
Children rehearse making excellent eye contact, connecting with new friends easily, and bringing out the best in their friends, skills that form balanced, contented adults.

OYC06 - Stimulating your Inner Creative Curiosity
Children learn to be curious about their surroundings while appreciating the beauty in all they see. By sparking inner creative curiosity, they develop an inquisitive mind and an interest in learning.

OYC07 - Your Parents Magically Know Best
Children come to understand that parental decisions are based on love and appreciation. Through parental love, children learn to become loving and caring adults.

OYC08 - Happy Mornings and Happy Bus Rides
Children rehearse waking up happy, getting dressed with excitement, eating a healthy breakfast, and completing all chores and morning rituals before going to school.

> *NOW is the perfect starting point for a bright and exciting future.*
> ~Patrick K Porter PhD

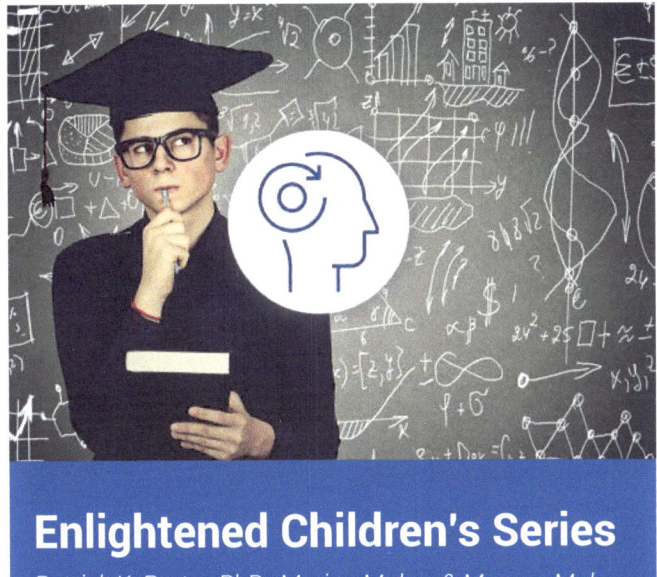

Enlightened Children's Series
Patrick K. Porter, PhD., Marina Mulac, & Morgan Mulac

Seven-year-old Marina Mulac and five-year-old Morgan Mulac, who have come to be known as the world's youngest marketers, were the inspiration behind this *Enlightened Children's* Series. When they met Dr. Patrick Porter, they had one question for him: Why had he created so many great visualizations for grown-ups and nothing for kids? Dr. Porter told the two little entrepreneurs that if they put on their thinking caps and helped him design a program for kids, together they could help children from around the globe to use their imaginative minds to become better people and help improve the world. This series that uses guided imagery, storytelling, and positive affirmations to help children see the world as a peaceful and harmonious place where everyone can win.

ESC01 - Building Optimism in Your Children
Optimists believe that people are inherently good and that most situations work out for the best. Your child will learn to see the good in every situation and how to be open to new experiences.

ESC02 - Developing Honesty as a Habit
Your child will realize that honesty is a way of communicating and acting truthfully.. This includes how he or she listens, speaks, and behaves around others.

ESC03 - Flying the Kite of Kindness
Your child will go to an imaginary park to fly a kite. While the wind takes hold of the kite, the child learns why kindness is a virtue and how to let his or her innate kindness shine for all to see.

ECS04 - Playing the Change Game
How children learn to adapt will influence their ability to cope with the stresses of our modern world. Your child will see change as a natural part of life and will learn the skills to master it.

ECS05 - Nurturing a Love of Learning
Your child will plant the seeds of curiosity that will develop into an excitement about learning new things.

ECS06 - Making Exercise Fun
When exercise becomes a way of life for your child, he or she will be spared the embarrassment and health risks associated with excess weight.

ECS07 - Practicing Patience
Patience involves persevering and remaining calm in the face of delay. Your child will discover that life unfolds over time and that their needs are met when the time is right.

ESC08 - Visualize Peace in the World
Your child will envision the peace he or she wants to see in the world by developing that peace within.

ESC09 - Respecting Yourself Respecting Others
Your child will gain a sense of self-worth and develop the ability to see the worth in others and to enjoy sharing their special gifts with the world.

ESC10 - Being the Light of Leadership
Your child will develop the skill of having a positive influence on others, and will learn to enlist the aid and support of others for accomplishing goals.

ESC11 - Bringing Compassion to the World
Compassion is often the key component to altruism and is embodied by the golden rule: Do unto others as you would have done to you. Your child will learn and rehearse this greatest of virtues.

ESC12 - Being the Gift of Love
One of Dr. Porter's mentors, the late Dr. Jerry DeShazo, was inspired to share *The Gift of Love* with the world. This is a spiritual poem that can be read a TheGiftofLove.com. Your child will learn this powerful visualization so that he or she can embody that gift in every word and deed.

ESC13 - Building Healthy Relationships
Your child will learn to identify with healthy relationships and will build that expectancy into developing healthy friendships. It will open communication between you and your child.

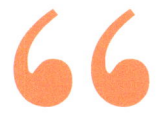

Our children are complete, just as God made them. We need to speak words of GREATNESS into our children. By speaking these words, we are growing seeds of GREATNESS.
~Dr. JoQueta Hayes Handy

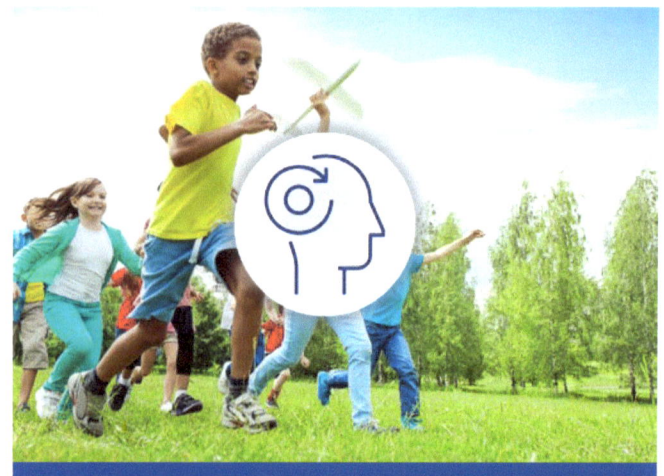

Consciousness - Children's Series
Cheree Porter

This series is designed to guide children to grow up into positive, productive, confident adults. The series includes sessions for being more optimistic and compassionate, as well as teaching the importance of exercise and eating right. These sessions range from 12-15 minutes, allowing your child just enough time to absorb the information being presented, without losing their attention.

MCS01 - Embracing Optimism
Here children learn to tap into their imaginations by meeting Will the Wizard, who guides them through the session and Katie the Caterpillar, who shares her story of life as a caterpillar.

MCS02 - Becoming Honest
Children learn to accept the power of the mind through the imagination, coming to understand that the imagination is a gift than can bring you what you want, and will help change you for the better.

MCS03 - Flying the Kite of Compassion
Demonstrating kindness to others goes a long way. Here children visualize a nice day at the park, with just enough breeze to keep the kite of compassion flying in the air. They then reminisce on a time when someone was kind t and they reciprocated that feeling to others.

MCS04 - Alchemy for Experiences
Alchemy is the art of changing one thing into something else, and we all know change is inevitable. Children will learn how to accept what they cannot change and to be comfortable when they outgrow situations.

MCS05 - Getting Back Your Love of Learning
Children will tap into their love of learning, which started when they were born. You will find that learning will come naturally to your child, no matter what is it you're trying to teach them.

MCS06 - Finding Fun Ways to Exercise
Many people dread exercising. This sessions is all about making exercise fun. No matter what type of exercise you choose to do, you will be able to relax and enjoy it.

MCS07 - Discovering the Joy of Being Patient
A lot of people lack patience. Your child will that even though they want something now, they are able to wait for it. Sometimes waiting for something makes it more special.

MCS08 - Peace Within Me, Peace Within the World
Creating peace within yourself is important. Your child will remember a time you he or she was calm and relaxed. Once you create peace within yourself, you can create peace within the world.

MCS09 - Building Respect for Yourself and Respect for Others
Your child will thank the different parts of his or her body for being there, and working as they should. Once you can thank your brain and body, you will be able to build respect for self and others.

MCS10 - Using Your Confidence to Lead Others
Here children step into the perspective of a leader and learn to use the same motivation they use to solve problems in life, and make something special happen in the world.

MCS11 - Love is the Law
Love is a beautiful thing. Your child will breathe in the feeling of love, and breathe out any negative feelings and learn to share this gift of love with the world.

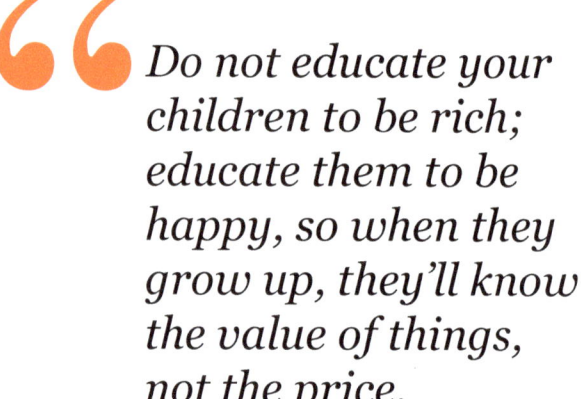

> *Do not educate your children to be rich; educate them to be happy, so when they grow up, they'll know the value of things, not the price.*
>
> ~Author Unknown

Christian

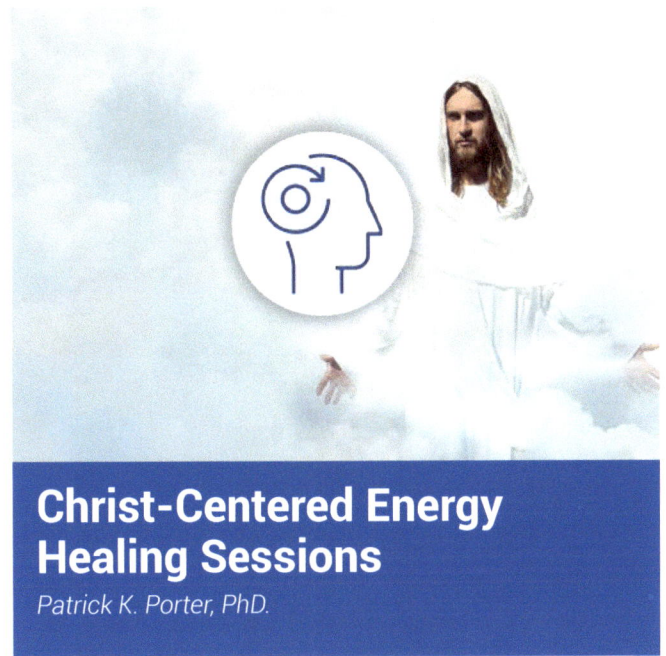

Christ-Centered Energy Healing Sessions
Patrick K. Porter, PhD.

This series is designed to allow you to focus more on Christ. You will learn that He is where your talents and gifts come from. You will learn about healing and how to call on the name of Jesus. After this series, you will be open to receive God's love and be ready to share God's message with the world. All you need to do is relax, and let Dr. Patrick Porter guide you through these Christ-centered sessions.

CCE-Demo - Christ Centered Energy Demo
In this demo session, you will learn to heal your body and purify your soul. Everything that happens through you, happens to you.

CCE01 - Being Thankful for Your Talents and Gifts of the Spirit
Many of us take our talents for granted. Here you will tap into your inner desire to share God's message with the world and learn to use your talents and gifts of the spirit.

CCE02 - Opening to Receive God's Love
James 5:16 is referenced in this session. It is often used when people gather together to pray for healing. You will focus on healing and allow the Christ-centered energy to flow from your mind.

CCE03 - Tap into the Power of the Name of Jesus
In this session, you will adjust the way you see the world. You are going to experience a peace, calm, and inner tranquility by tapping into the power of the name of Jesus.

CCE04 - Gratitude, Acceptance, and Clarity in Christ
Here you will learn that all healing comes from a divine source, and you will allow healing to move through your entire body in order to find clarity in Christ.

CCE05 - Forgiveness, your Key to Acceptance
You may find it hard to forgive. You will learn that forgiveness is your key to acceptance. You will be able to let go and let God.

CCE06 - Healing the Body, Purifying your Soul
You will learn to call on the Lord for help in healing your body. Once your body has been healed, you will then purify your soul.

CCE07 - Be Ready to Share God's Message with the World
You may have reservations when it comes to sharing God's message, but with this session you will let go and share God's message willingly and freely.

Peak Performance - Balancing Your Life in Christ
Dr. Randy Shepard

This series is designed to achieve peak performance by balancing your life in Christ. Dr. Randy Shepard will guide you and show you how to balance your life in Christ, as well as manage stress, while incorporating the word of God.

PPBL01 - Balancing Your Life in Christ
Balance is everything. When you have it, you feel calm, grounded, and motivated. Experience the life-transforming word of God and a scriptural remedy to build balance back into your life.

PPBL02 - Health and Wellness
Dr. Shepard will share the wisdom of God's word, and the simple techniques used since the beginning of time to build and maintain a healthy, vibrant life.

Gospel Meditation - GV01
Amanda White

Amanda White will guide you through a gospel meditation where you will realize that you are powerful, and you will learn to be strong in the Lord.

Christian Weight Loss
Christopher Wallace

CWL01 - Start Each Day with Faith, Love, and Thankfulness
You will allow the peace, love, and joy of God that passes all understanding to be with you during this session. You will learn to be happy, healthy, and at your ideal, natural weight.

Dentistry

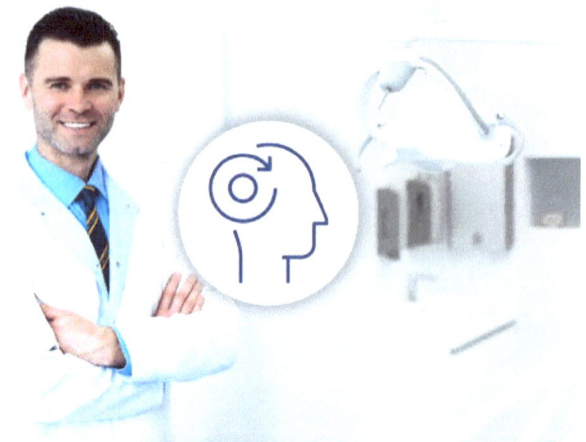

Stress-Free Dentistry Series
Patrick K. Porter, PhD.

Whether you get sweaty palms at the thought of a dentist's drill, hyperventilate the moment you lay eyes on a dental syringe, or get butterflies in your stomach before going to the dentist, this program can benefit you. We are all born with certain fears that protect us, such as the fear of falling and the fear of loud noises. Fear stops us from doing dangerous things. The purpose of this series is to put fear in its proper perspective so you can have a relaxed experience at every dental visit.

SFD01 - Relax and Control the Dental Experience
You will learn a simple technique that will have you visualizing a pleasant visit to your dentist's office as well as releasing emotions tied to any negative experiences with dental procedures.

SFD02 - Mental Rehearsal for Instant Relaxation
This relaxing session uses a distraction technique that will eliminate anxiety and fear. Dentistry may not ever be fun for you, but it can be a relaxed and comfortable experience.

SFD03 – Eliminate False Beliefs & Build Self-Confidence
You will explore beliefs about dentistry, and eliminate those that are impacting you negatively. You will build the self-confidence necessary to comfortably handle any dental appointment.

SFD04 – Setting Expectations and Eliminating Dental Anxiety
This session will help you quickly build your self-esteem and enhance your assertiveness. You will begin acting as your own advocate, asking the right questions.

SFD05 - Control What You Think and Feel
In this session you will master the art of singular thinking, allowing you to create a state of relaxation where you can control the sensations in your body by controlling your thoughts.

Diabetes

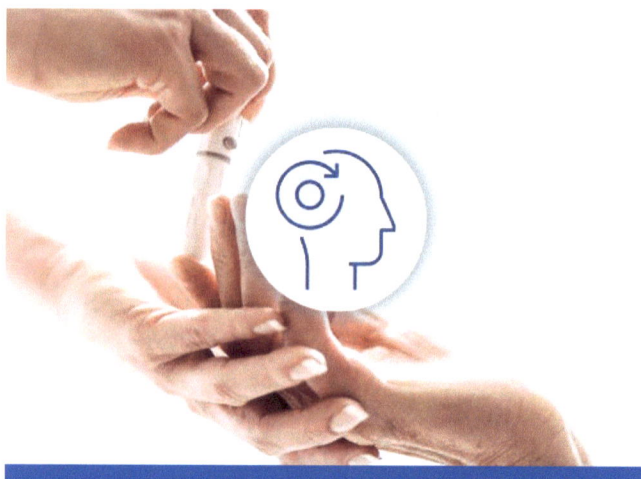

Diabetes Active Lifestyle Program
Patrick K. Porter, PhD & Owen Durkin

Diabetes affects 26 million Americans, making it likely you know someone who has diabetes, or perhaps you have diabetes. Now Dr. Patrick Porter has partnered with Owen Durkin, a researcher and father of a child with diabetes, to help you manage the stress of this lifestyle disease. It is said, "You don't have to like diabetes, you just have to get along with it," and that is just what you are going to do. Follow these 7 transformative sessions and make the management and navigation of your diabetes easier.

IMPORTANT! This series is intended to address habits and lifestyle choices and should never be used in place of professional medical or mental health intervention.

DAL01 - Activate Your Daily Plan for an Active Lifestyle
This session will show you how your daily management plan is the key to a complication-free lifestyle. People with diabetes (PWDs) can learn to enjoy a healthy, complication-free life, all you need is a plan!

DAL02 – Stimulate Your Daily Commitment
You will learn the keys to preventing the onset of disruptive symptoms, increasing your quality of life both physically and emotionally.

DAL03 – Being Proactive in Your Daily Diabetes Management
You will become proactive in managing your diabetes. Frequent monitoring allows you to treat fluctuations in blood glucose in a timely manner, and to avoid these side effects.

DAL04 - Personal Choice - Your Commitment to a Complication-Free Life
Implementing a strategy comes down to personal choice and commitment to a complication-free life. You will learn to use some powerful tools to help you refine your personal management plan.

DAL05 – Consistency - Your Key to Successful Diabetes Relief
The key to successful management is consistency, which you will mentally rehearse during this session. You will become more consistent with managing diabetes, while maintaining a positive attitude.

DAL06 – Doing Your Part to Keep Blood Sugar Level
You will learn the kind of discipline needed to stay on the course of good disease management. You will learn to stay calm when challenged by circumstances that otherwise may overwhelm you.

DAL07 – Eliminate Failure as an Option
You may feel like diabetes is a losing battle. This session provides an alternative to the endless strain of fighting this battle. You will begin to reclaim your life, be active and symptom-free for years to come.

Fasting for Health

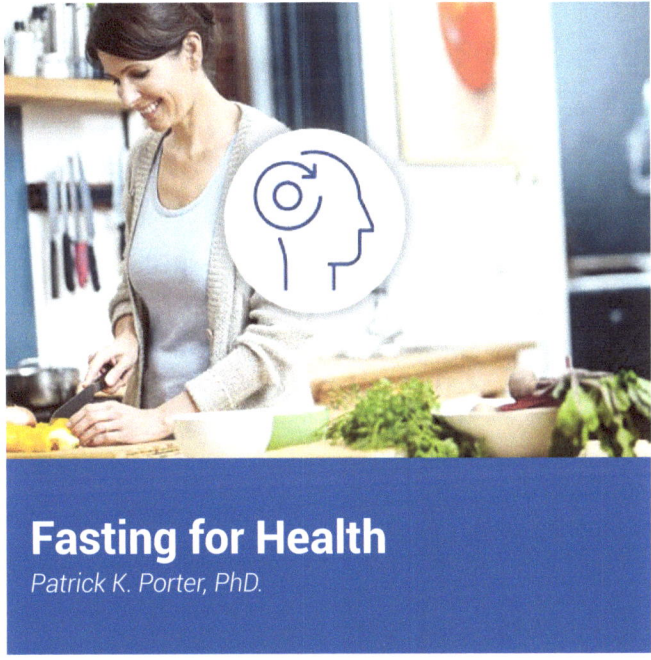

Fasting for Health
Patrick K. Porter, PhD.

FFH01 - Fasting for Health
Learn why fasting is both natural and healthy and how to do it safely and effectively. At the same time, you'll get motivated to succeed.

Gluten-Free Lifestyle

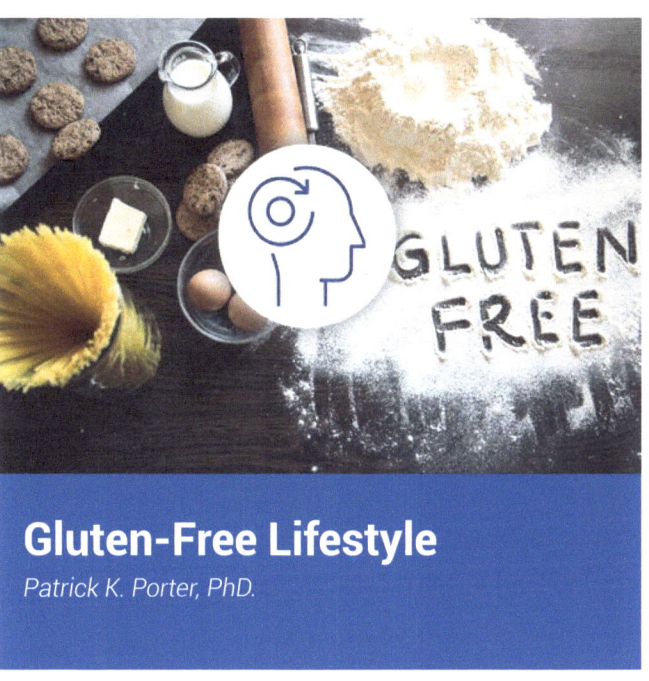

Gluten-Free Lifestyle
Patrick K. Porter, PhD.

Health experts from all sides of the nutrition spectrum, including weight loss specialists, bariatric physicians, and dietitians, are talking about the health benefits of a gluten-free diet, especially considering the escalating number of people being diagnosed with celiac disease and gluten sensitivity. A gluten-free diet can have a variety of health benefits, such as eliminating digestive problems, improving cholesterol levels, lowering blood sugar, and increasing energy. Even people who don't have a gluten problem are opting for a gluten-free lifestyle because of the health benefits. For example, on a gluten-free diet, you would likely eat more fruits and vegetables, because these are readily available food sources that are naturally gluten-free. A gluten-free diet can also help ward off viruses and germs, because many of the replacement foods are full of antioxidants and essential vitamins and minerals. Needless to say, a gluten-free diet is a worthwhile endeavor, and this BrainTap series will help make your transition to gluten-free easy and fun!

GFL01 Stimulate Your Metabolism - Go Gluten-Free
It's never easy making a life change if stress is an overriding factor. Seeking out healthy alternatives will have your energy improving, and your waistline rapidly returning to normal.

GFL02 Unlock Your Body's Health - Live Gluten-Free
You will train your brain to avoid negative carbohydrates, the worst gas producing foods. You will focus on a gluten-free diet low in refined carbohydrates, so you can feel better and get healthier.

GFL03 Visualize Your Gluten-Free Lifestyle
You will create a timeline for becoming gluten-free.. You will begin noticing a calming effect on your nervous system, which will help eliminate nighttime cravings.

GFL04 Stress-Free, Gluten-Free
You will learn a bulletproof method for saying no to gluten products. Your waistline will return to normal naturally, and as the discomfort in your colon is relieved, you will start to enjoy life again.

GFL05 Shopping Gluten-Free
Eliminate confusion while you visualize enjoying fresh fruits and vegetables. You will focus on fat burning, healthier bones, and freedom from joint pain.

GFL06 Eating Out Gluten-Free
You will learn a technique where you can look over any menu and easily choose gluten-free foods. Your self-esteem will soar as you realize that you are worth the time, energy, and effort of staying gluten-free.

GFL07 Gluten-Free Travel (Theater of the Mind)
You will learn to succeed in any environment, instead of counting on failure, and will be able to plan ahead with gluten-free foods on the top of your priority list.

Grief

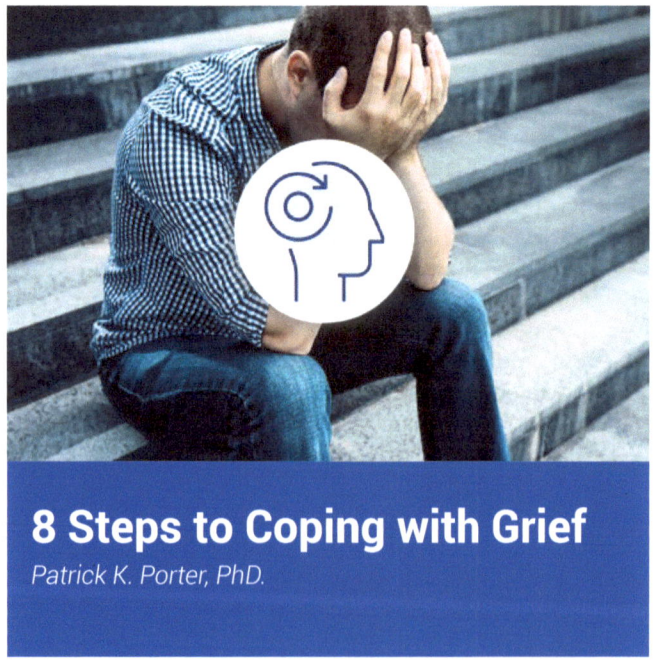

8 Steps to Coping with Grief
Patrick K. Porter, PhD.

No one wants to experience the loss of a loved one, however it affects everyone at some point or another. Once grief hits, it may feel unbearable, however you can get through this difficult time, which is exactly what this series is designed to do. You will learn an 8-step process that will help you acknowledge the impact of the loss, begin healing, and make peace with what happened. You will also learn how to regain your happiness while still cherishing the memories of your loved one.

GR01 - Acknowledge the Impact of Loss
Numbness is a normal reaction to an immediate loss, and should not be confused with lack of caring. You will acknowledge the impact of the loss so that denial and disbelief will diminish, opening the door to the natural grieving process.

GR02 - Eliminate the Persistent Thoughts of Guilt
People can become preoccupied about how things could have gone differently. This session will help you properly move through this process, so that intense feelings of remorse or guilt will not interfere with the healing process.

GR03 - Regain Your Sense of Self
This stage of grief occurs in some people after realizing the extent of the loss. Signs may include sleep and appetite disturbances, lack of energy, and crying spells. This session will help you get back to living a full and productive life.

GR04 - Making Peace with the Process of Life
Anger can stem from a feeling of abandonment through a loved one's death. You may sometimes feel anger toward a higher power or life in general. This session will gently process this anger and lift the weight of helplessness from your shoulders.

GR05 - Accept the Healing and Put the Past into Perspective
In time, you will come to terms with various feelings and accept the fact that the loss has occurred. This session moves the acceptance process along and sets the stage for healing by integrating the loss into your set of life experiences.

GR06 - Building a New Perspective on Grief
This session will help make your day-to-day living calmer and more organized. As your life begins to settle into place, your physical symptoms will lessen and your sadness will begin to lift, letting you focus on the happy experiences you had with your loved one.

GR07 - Daily Problem Solving for Health and Happiness
As you become more functional, your mind starts working again, and you will find yourself seeking realistic solutions to problems posed by life without your loved one. This session will help you reconstruct yourself and your life.

GR08 - Building Balance in Every Situation
This final session will help ensure that you learn to accept and deal with the reality of your situation. You will, once again, anticipate the good times to come, and even find joy in the experience of living, while always cherishing the happiness you shared with your loved one.

Health

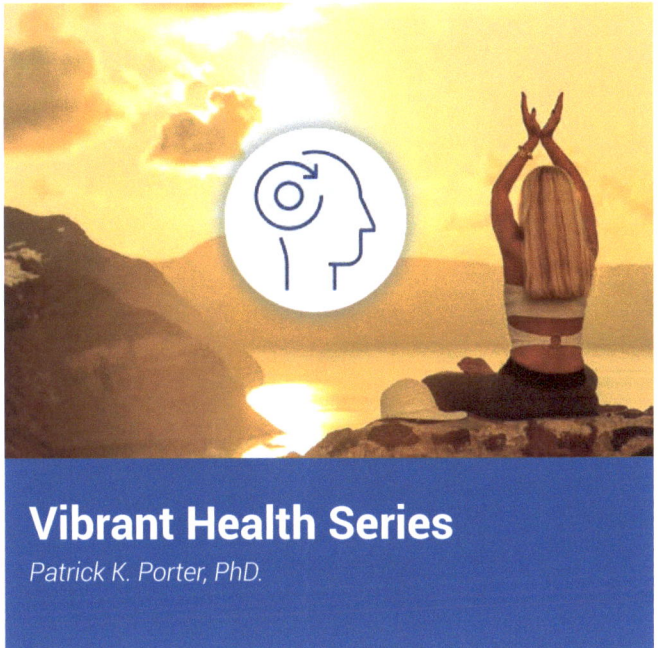

Vibrant Health Series
Patrick K. Porter, PhD.

Of all the cells in your body, more than 50,000 will die and be replaced with new cells, all in the time it took you to read this sentence! Your body is the vehicle you have been given for the journey of your life. How you treat your body determines how it will treat you. Dr. Patrick Porter (PhD) will show you how you can recharge and energize your body, mind, and spirit. This series is for people who are looking for more than good health; it's for those who will settle for nothing less than vibrant health!

VH01 - Staying Focused in the Present
You will benefit by reducing negative feelings such as regret, worry, or anxiety, which only add stress to the body, which makes you more susceptible to disease.

VH02 - Visualize a Heart-Healthy Lifestyle
To protect your heart, you need a plan that includes movement, a healthy diet, and a positive mental attitude. You'll find smiling even easier now that you are actively protecting the health of your heart.

VH03 - Exercise Just Do It!
Many people hate exercising. In this session you will learn about exercising, and the human body. You will begin to exercise to help you live a longer, happier, and healthier life.

VH04 - Unlocking the Healing Force of Positive Thoughts
Negative thoughts can severely impact your health. You will learn a visualization technique that will help you quickly catch negative thoughts and turn them into a positive affirmation.

VH05 - Planning a Healthy Diet for Vibrant Health
You will visualize a healthy lifestyle where the live foods are appealing to you, and the processed and fast foods are a turn-off. You will learn to provide your body with the high quality fuel it needs.

VH06 - Train Your Brain to Give You Adequate Rest
You will be taken through a full sleep cycle, and you will begin engaging in the REM sleep pattern to begin healing and rejuvenating your body.

VH07 - Problem Solving For Vibrant Health
The brain creates unhealthy neuro-chemicals whenever you are focused on problems. By placing your attention on solutions, you encourage your brain to create the healthy neuro-chemicals that make you feel good.

VH08 - Supercharge Your Memory & Concentration
You will learn simple tips for improving your everyday memory of names, addresses, events, and whatever else you wish to remember. You will gain confidence in knowing that your memory is getting stronger and your brain is staying healthy.

VH09 - Surround Yourself With a Great Support System
This session will give you tactful ways to receive support from people who will care for, love, respect, and appreciate you as you reach your goal of vibrant health.

> *The brain is the greatest pharmacy on earth, capable of producing 30,000 different neuro-chemicals in a moment's notice.*
>
> **~Patrick K Porter PhD**

5 Simple Steps to Optimal Health

The most dangerous health epidemic we face today is *Super-Stress*. This epidemic is a result of the fast-paced lifestyle in this new era of total connectivity. Stress often manifests in disorders such as ADHD, obesity, diabetes, insomnia, headaches, and high blood pressure to name but a few.

When we're under stress, our bodies pump out adrenaline and cortisol, an effect of the *fight-or-flight* response, which is the mechanism our bodies employ to keep us safe from injury or attack. Problems arise when the daily onslaught of stress leaves us stuck in this highly-aroused state where all resources are focused on survival.

Sadly, we've become so accustomed to this *super-stress* lifestyle that we don't even realize the damage it's doing to our mental and physical health. Since we can't escape the fast-paced, high-tech lifestyle of the 21st Century, we must learn new ways to deal with the stresses of life to prevent it from causing problems for us, both physically and psychologically.

Our bodies must return to a state of homeostasis (balance) for recovery, repair and healing to take place, but few people know how to do that. Keep reading, though, because our **5 Simple Steps to Optimal Health** couldn't be easier.

TIP #1: BREATHE DEEPLY
Deep breathing is one of the best ways to lower stress because when you breathe deeply, it sends a message to your brain to calm the body. The stress responses that are so detrimental to our health—such as increased heart rate, increased hormone production and high blood pressure—all decrease as you breathe deeply to relax. Just a few minutes of deep breathing can calm you and put the body back into recovery mode. For this reason, every audio session in our library includes deep, relaxing, guided breathing designed to bring your body to ultimate relaxation.

Recommended BrainTap session:
SR01- Create Your Enchanted Forest for Stress Reduction

TIP #2 - FOCUS ON THE MOMENT
When you are stressed and anxious, you're most likely dwelling on a past event or a future one. You're worried about what comes next or regretting something you've already done. This can cause immense amounts of stress from which our bodies need recovery time.

One way to lessen this type of stress is to bring yourself back to the moment. If you're walking, feel the sensation of your legs moving your body. If you're eating, focus on the taste, the smell, the sensation of the food you're consuming. If you're relaxing, be mindful of the heaviness of your limbs and the deep, rhythmic sound of your breathing. Rather than seeing only the negatives, focusing on the moment offers you a space to think differently about stress and respond in a more appropriate manner without past regrets or future worries.

Recommended BrainTap session: *SR04 - Putting Future Events into Perspective*

TIP # 3- REFRAME THE SITUATION
When we are stressed or overwhelmed, it may seem impossible to find a positive thought, but it's not as hard as you think. When you reframe a situation, you're simply looking at the same situation in a new way that highlights the possibilities. Viewing our stressors as opportunities can help us stop feeling trapped and reduce the physical effects of stress on our bodies almost immediately.

So how can you reframe any situation?
1. **Look at what is actually stressing you**
2. **Consider what you can change, if anything, about the situation**
3. **Look for the positives**
4. **Find the humor**

Recommended BrainTap session:
SR05 - Reducing Uncertainty and Doubt

TIP #4 - KEEP YOUR PROBLEMS IN PERSPECTIVE
We tend to stay in stress mode when we focus too much on a specific problem. It's important to remind ourselves of the positives in our lives—we woke up this morning; we can see; we can walk; we have family and friends to support us. It might seem a little silly at first, but the next time you're feeling stressed, consciously make the effort to think about the things you're grateful for. This can be a surprisingly easy way to reduce the stress in your life.

Recommended BrainTap session:
SR 06 - Eliminate Negative Thinking

TIP #5 - PRACTICE MINDFUL MEDITATION AND VISUALIZATION
By practicing mindful meditation and visualization, you can achieve the **relaxation response,** a physical state of deep rest that changes the physical and emotional responses to stress. Once you enter the relaxation response, the brain sends out neurochemicals that neutralize the effects of stress on the body, allowing you to change your reactions to the stressful events going on around you. The sessions offered in the BrainTap Library are designed to help you reach the relaxation response. In 20 relaxing minutes a day you can reduce or eliminate brain fog and negative mind chatter, have more energy, relax and develop positive sleep habits, rid yourself of unwanted habits and behaviors, gain memory and focus, and improve the quality of your life.

Recommended BrainTap session:
SR10 - Developing Spontaneous Relaxation

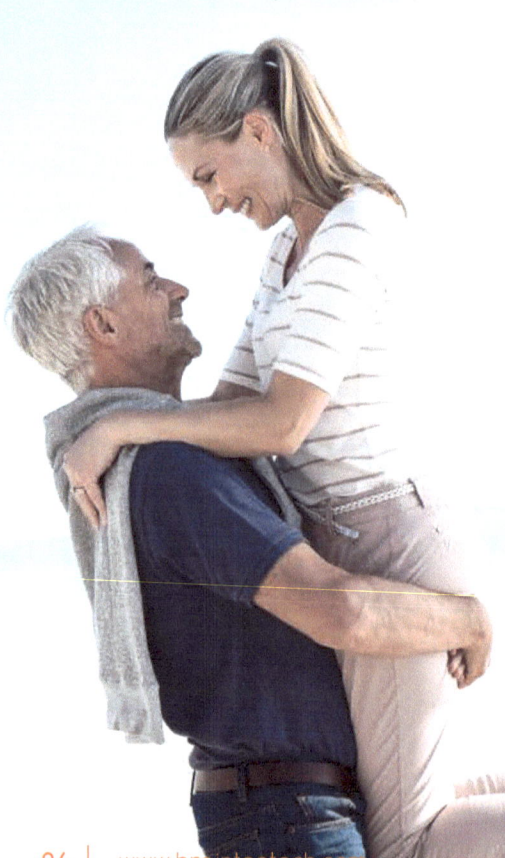

Heart Health

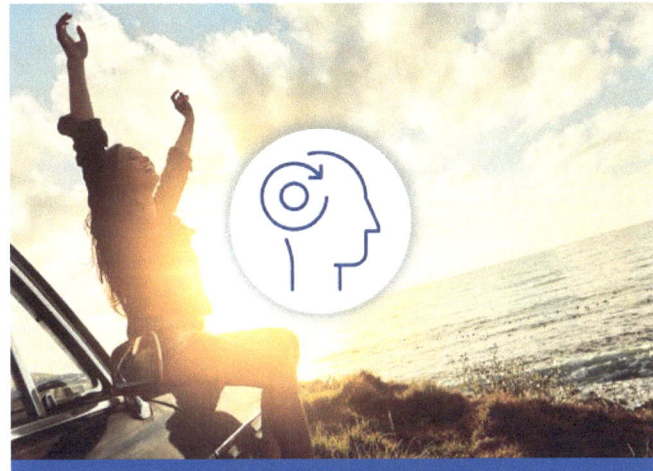

Heart Health
Patrick K. Porter, Ph.D.
Inspired by the principles of Dr. Michael Irving's Twelve Wisdoms to a Healthy Heart

Adversities and life challenges can be viewed as burdens or as gifts. A heart attack or diagnosis of heart disease is a dramatic wake up call. Dr. Porter and Dr. Irving want you to see your diagnosis as the gift that it is—the opportunity to create a heart-healthy lifestyle and a brand new you!

While watching a nail-biting Stanley Cup hockey game, Dr. Irving experienced a life-threatening heart attack. The reality of his mortality brought into perspective his busy lifestyle and unhealthy habits. So profound were the positive changes he made in his life, it led his rehab supervisor to say that in twenty-five years at one of North America's largest cardiac clinics she had never before seen such dramatic improvement across such a broad range of measures. By following Dr. Irving's lead, you too can be inspired to reverse heart disease and enjoy a life you love. You will begin by internalizing Dr. Irving's "Twelve Wisdoms to a Healthy Heart" which include: 1) Taking Charge 2) Family and Friends 3) A Health Care Team 4) Medicines and Supplements 5) Visualization 6) Heart Healthy Food 7) Exercise for Life 8) Stress Reduction 9) Listening to Your Heart 10) Harmony and Balance 11) Meditation and Relaxation 12) A Spiritual Connection.

IMPORTANT! This series is intended to address habits and lifestyle choices while enhancing spiritual faith and should never be used in place of professional medical or mental health intervention.

HHL01 – Gifts Found in Accepting the Challenges to Your Heart
A heart crisis can be frightening, but it can also make you feel grateful to be alive. This first session helps you define resolutions and motivates you to take action. These changes will have you on your way to a vibrant life.

HHL02 – Take Charge with a Strong Heart
You will take ownership of your health and be the central director of your success. You will become confident in your knowledge of heart health, and become ready to make the decisions that fulfill your goals.

HHL03 – Opening the Heart to Family and Friends
After a cardiac crisis, you may feel isolated from family and friends. In this session you will learn to accept gestures of genuine love and concern, so you will be well on your way to healing.

HHL04 – Gathering a Health Care Team for Your Heart
You will learn to take full advantage of the wisdom your healthcare team offers. You will feel empowered to ask questions and gather the information you need for an optimal recovery.

HHL05 – Medicines and Supplements for Heart Health and Recovery
Medicines, herbs, and remedies can help you manage and reverse heart disease. You will direct the power of your mind and body to work with your medicines and supplements for ideal effectiveness.

HHL06 – The Power of Visualization for Heart Health
This session brings the mind, body, and heart together to create and enhance positive feelings. You will make the mind/body connection for healing, making positive life choices easily and naturally.

HHL07 – Heart Healthy Food for Life
Reinforce what your body already knows; fresh vegetables and whole foods make your heart and arteries healthy and vital. You will visualize your food as healing medicine while you plan, shop for, and cook your heart-healthy meals.

HHL08 – Strengthen the Heart with Exercise for Life
You will gain positive images of your physical fitness, learning that regular exercise helps clear the body of stress, builds muscle, strengthens the heart, and creates energy and vitality throughout the day.

HHL09 – Stress Reduction to Calm the Heart
You will uncover what is at the root of your stress. This session will open you up to the tranquility already present within you.

HHL10 – Listening to Your Heart
If you are feeling a heavy heart, simply listen to this session and learn to lighten it. Your heart will guide you toward your passions in life; all you have to do is listen.

HHL11 – Harmony and Balance for a Quiet Heart
This session will help you find ways to ground yourself, have variety in your life, find time for pleasure, manage your work life, and approach life activities with mindfulness.

HHL12 – Meditation and Relaxation for a Peaceful Heart
You will learn to achieve the relaxation response, a powerful key to releasing the natural healing forces of the brain and body. You will gain inner strength and recognize that your life is abundant.

HHL13 – Spiritual Connections from the Heart
A life-death confrontation of a cardiac incident can be a frightening. This session will inspire you to realize you can have a better and more fulfilling life. You will increase your thoughts of meaning, purpose, and a higher power.

Irritable Bowel Syndrome

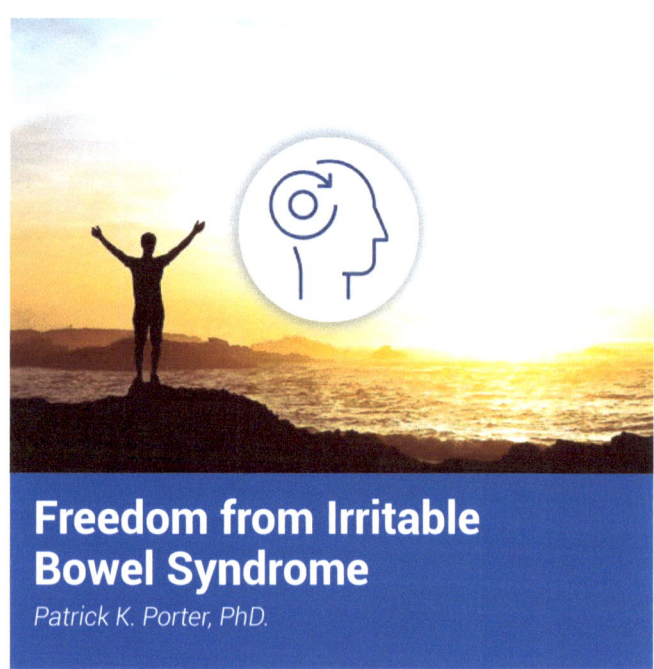

Freedom from Irritable Bowel Syndrome
Patrick K. Porter, PhD.

Irritable Bowel Syndrome (IBS) is when a person's intestines squeeze too hard or not hard enough and cause food to move too quickly or too slowly through the digestive tract. However, it is believed that most cases of IBS are a side-effect of the stress response, making it more of a thinking problem than a physical one. Patrick K. Porter, Ph.D was first asked to help with IBS back in the 1980s when a client showed him a series of magazine articles about how United Kingdom doctors regularly refer IBS sufferers to therapists who practice relaxation and visualization techniques, which started him on a quest to help his clients with this uncomfortable problem. This series was the result of that quest.

IMPORTANT! This series is intended to address habits and lifestyle choices while enhancing spiritual faith and should never be used in place of professional medical or mental health intervention.

IBS01 -- Mental Tips on Controlling Your IBS Symptoms
This foundation session teaches you to take the time to reduce your stress and apprehension. You will become familiar with the mind/body connection and learn to eliminate the emotional triggers that make you feel out of control.

IBS02 -- Being Physically & Mentally Balanced
Eating foods that make you feel worse will only add to the stress associated with IBS. This session helps you manage IBS symptoms by helping you understand the benefits of allowing both mind and body to work together toward the goal of relief.

IBS03 – Stress Buster - Your Key to IBS Relief
Most IBS sufferers find that symptoms worsen when they travel, attend social events, or change their daily routine. You will learn the relaxation response that will instantly put you back in control.

IBS04 -- Using Your Mind to Regulate Your Body
Your mind can be your worst enemy at times. This session will show you how to use the power of suggestion to imagine having a normal bowel movement. You will learn to regulate your body with proper diet and relaxation.

IBS05 – Staying True to Your Body for IBS Support
Food sensitivity can be a major cause of IBS. These mental exercises will help you avoid the foods that cause the problem to worsen. You will also use visualization to increase your fiber, which improves how the intestines work.

IBS06 -- Tips on controlling IBS for a Healthy Life
You will learn a technique that will eliminate stress and help you stay focused on healthy living. You will build a support system including your health care provider, and stay mentally prepared for success by exercising, relaxing, or meditating.

> *When you trust in your mind, it will be true to you.*
> ~Patrick K Porter PhD

Learning

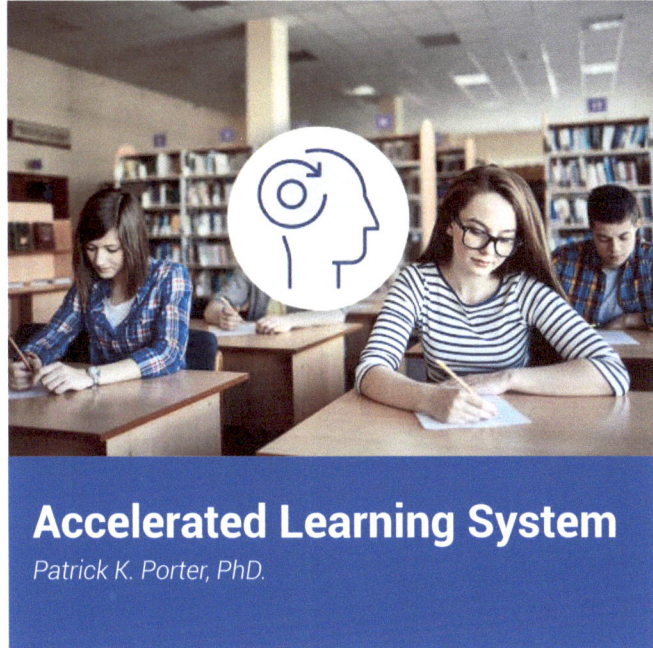

Accelerated Learning System
Patrick K. Porter, PhD.

Whether you are an honor student or just having difficulty taking a test, this breakthrough learning system will help you overcome learning challenges and accelerate your current skill level. Imagine doubling your reading speed while improving your memory. Sit back, relax, and allow your mind to organize your life, while you build your self-confidence, and earn better grades with the complete learning system.

ALS01 - Setting Goals for Learning Success
Successful students are those who have an outcome or ultimate goal in mind. With this session you will learn the secrets of goal setting, experience a boost in motivation, and see your self-confidence in the classroom soar.

ALS02 – Being an Optimistic Thinker
Henry Ford once said, "Whether you think you can, or you think you can't, you are right." It all starts with attitude. Discover ways of breaking through to your optimistic mind that will help you to think, act, and respond with a positive nature.

ALS03 - Six Steps to Using Your Perfect Memory
Memory issues affect plenty of people today. You will discover creative ways to access and recall the information you need as you need it. You will benefit by relaxing your mind, using the six steps that activate a perfect memory.

ALS04 - Secrets for Increasing Your Reading Speed
Slow reading can be frustrating, however, our minds absorb every word on a page as soon as we scan it. This session features ways to break through the barriers that prevent you from reading at the speed and comprehension level you desire.

ALS05 - Using the Tricks of Highly Successful Students
Discover the best-kept secrets of successful students, and how to apply them in your own life. You will soon discover that if someone else can do what you want to do, you can model what that person is doing, and master it for yourself.

ALS06 - Problem Solving with Your Creative Mind
Follow in the footsteps of great thinkers such as Einstein and step into the realm of infinite possibility where imagination and creativity are limitless. You will solve your everyday problems with solutions found in the present and future.

ALS07 - Activate Your Hidden Talents
Your skills and talents go beyond your one-dimensional IQ (Intelligence Quotient). You will relax, and activate the different stages of intelligence within you. You will become a person of intellect on multiple levels.

ALS08 - Demonstrate Self-Confidence in Learning
Concentration is key to learning. You will discover a powerful concentration exercise that will unlock your true confidence. Once unlocked, you can succeed at anything you put your mind to.

ALS09 - Speak with Passion and Power
You might not have been born a public speaker, but with these foolproof methods to activate your other-than-conscious mind, you will have the power and skill to speak freely, easily, and clearly, whenever you're presenting.

ALS10 - End Self-Sabotage at School
A lot of issues you face in the classroom come from self-sabotage. With this session, you will eliminate old patterns and unleash your ultimate power to manifest your dreams in and out of the classroom.

ALS11 – Finishing Assignments and Projects
Completing assignments in a timely manner is one of the most common concerns in school. In You will tap into the unseen power of your other-than-conscious mind to get organized and efficiently complete any project.

ALS12 - Turning Homework Procrastination into Motivation
This module will have you practicing the eight steps to transform procrastination into motivation. You will have more fun completing your homework, or starting a new project, than you ever dreamed possible.

ALS13 – The Power of Affirmations in the Classroom
Encouragement in the classroom can help make or break your success. You will discover how the right words can create a powerful mental image of you in the classroom that will lead you to your educational goals.

Life Improvement

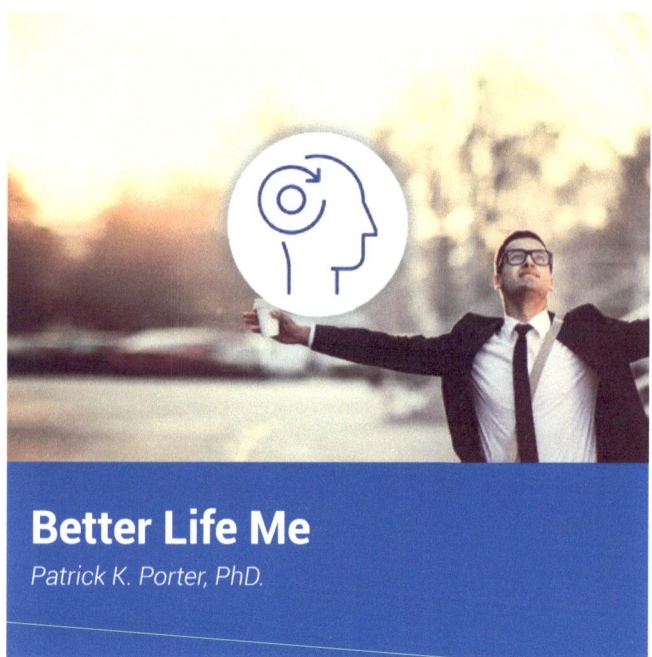

Better Life Me
Patrick K. Porter, PhD.

The Better Life Me series is dedicated to those wanting to live a better life. During these sessions you will learn the importance of balancing your health, finances, relationships, among other areas of your life. If you've been looking to make improvements in your life, this is the series for you. Just sit back, relax, and allow Dr. Patrick Porter show you what it takes to create a better life for yourself.

BLM01 - Committing To Your Balanced Life
Learn how to integrate the 8 essential segments of the Wheel of Life. You will learn how to create good health, incorporate strategies to build wealth, and take control of your finances, just to name a few.

BLM02 - Health and Wellbeing Visualization
Learn how to create a timeline for change that will have you eating and drinking the most nutritious foods available. You will learn how to make that mind/body connection to help you maintain your healthiest you.

BLM03 - Wealth and Finances Visualization
Discover why managing your wealth and finances starts with the way you manage your thoughts. You will learn the secrets of the wealth builders, and how to master your thoughts, and master your finances.

BLM04 - Relationships Visualization
You will use your creative mind to relate to your family and friends. It will be natural for you to be easy going and accepting, and let others have their own opinion, without wanting to win them over.

BLM05 - Lifestyle Visualization
Making lifestyle changes can seem difficult. You will work through any self-judgement, and develop the simple balanced life that will bring you the greatest joy.

BLM06 - Personal Growth Visualization
You will learn to listen to your heart. You will experience the joy of negative beliefs melting away, leaving you free to do something new.

BLM07 - Career Visualization
Learn to unlock your true potential that will work to shift your attitude. You will learn how to use your strengths to help you get from where you are to where you want to go in the safest, and quickest amount of time.

BLM08 - Environment Visualization
You will learn to appreciate nature's gift. You will create the re-connection with the world that will empower you to take an active role to really understand what the environment means to you.

BLM09 - Spirituality Visualization
Learn to understand the consciousness that is you. You will explore your intuition, and allow the happiness of your spirit to show up in your life in ways that you can't imagine with inner resources you didn't know you have.

BLM10 – You Can Be The Change
Let the Wheel of Life concepts to guide you through exercises that will put your life into perspective. You will unleash the power of thought and action, and strive to balance the 8 areas of your life.

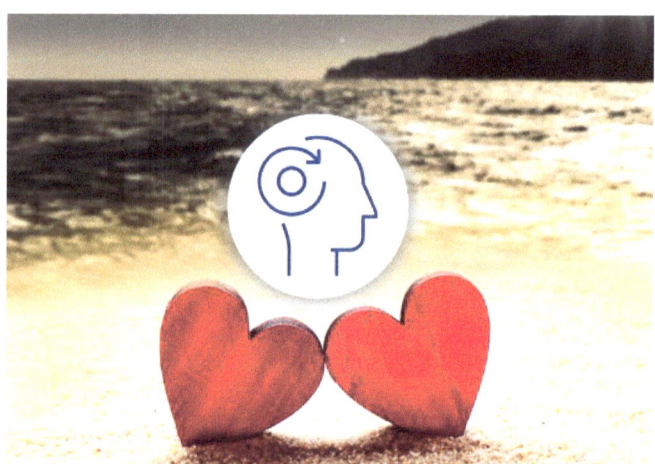

Finding Love and Building Winning Relationships
Patrick K. Porter, Ph.D. & Michael Irving, Ph.D.

Winning at dating involves building relationship skills that you can apply to the world of dating and romance. With Dr. Michael Irving's powerful techniques, and Dr. Patrick Porter's guiding voice, this program provides you a step-by-step plan for creating a winning attitude and positive outlook, the key life skills needed to succeed at dating and in romantic relationships. Dr. Porter

& Dr. Irving understand that finding a date is never easy, but you can increase your odds dramatically by harnessing the right attitude, developing the habit of positive self-talk, and changing any negative beliefs you have created around dating.

WR00 - 10-Minute Preview Session: Building Winning Relationships
This introductory session is designed to help you awaken the self-confidence within you, so you can start feeling comfortable and secure in responding to the dating opportunities presented to you.

WR01 - Taking Charge of Your Dating Success
You will see how the dating game is at your door just waiting for you to embrace it. As you take charge of your personal approach to dating, you will find yourself trying new things to look and feel better.

WR02 - Overcoming Shyness
You will eliminate the shyness that inhibits, or even paralyzes you from taking up new relationships. You will create a new you with radiant self-confidence, helping you strike up conversations, and hold the attention of others.

WR03 - Freedom From Criticism ... It's In Your Power
You will acquire resiliency, and learn to rise above criticism. When you know you are good enough for yourself, you are naturally good enough for others.

WR04 - Increase Your Attraction Through Confident Flirting
The confidence you display is the key factor in successful flirting. You will feel confident knowing that successful flirting is a natural response, and begin comfortably sending signals that you are interested and available.

WR05 - Letting Go of Fear and Visualizing Dating Success
You are going to visualize a successful date, with someone you like and who likes you, as the new you who enjoys simple, casual, carefree, and fun experiences.

WR06 - Finding a Date In The Expansive World Around You
You will integrate looking for dates with a positive attitude into your everyday social routine. You will know that there are opportunities just waiting to present a special someone in your life.

Life Improvement

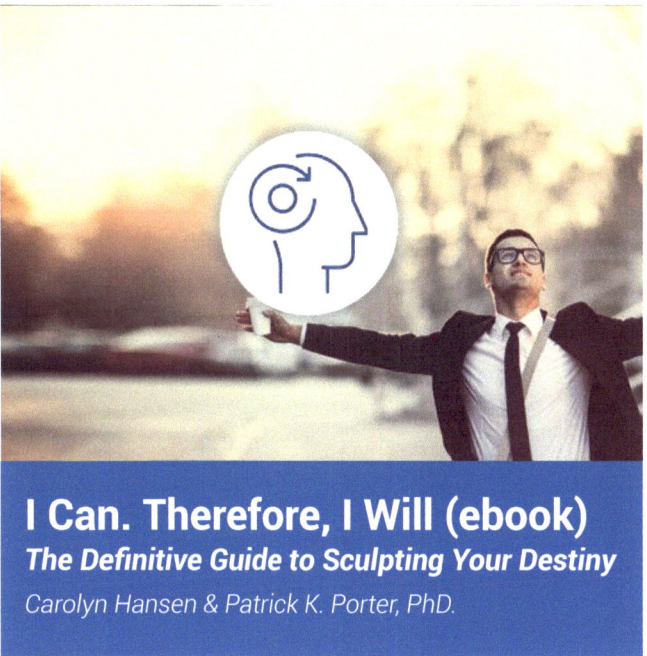

I Can. Therefore, I Will (ebook)
The Definitive Guide to Sculpting Your Destiny
Carolyn Hansen & Patrick K. Porter, PhD.

Reading and assimilating the wisdom found in *I Can. Therefore I Will* is the first step to a rewarding and fulfilling life. As you devour the content in this breakthrough ebook, it will reveal the secrets behind manifesting your dreams.f.

The Goal Setting Workbook
This goal setting workbook breaks down the most difficult parts of goal setting into easy baby steps. It will keep you accountable to your word and help you internalize positive daily habits.

Here's what you'll discover in this ebook and workbook:
- Exercises on what you did great last year and how to propel this year
- Set an intention to increase your focus on certain areas of attention
- Resolve to change certain bad habits and take on good ones
- Set definite goals and propel your success
- Harness the power of specificity
- How to set goals from your heart so you will succeed at all costs
- How to break them all down into baby steps so everything is achievable
- And more...

Dr. Patrick Porter (PhD) has designed a series that will help you super-charge the core message in *I Can, Therefore I Will*. These sessions are designed to train the subconscious to work in harmony with your conscious mind. Check out the details on what each audio will teach you!

iCan01 - Building Your New Thought Generator
As you learn that thoughts are more powerful than things because thoughts create things, you will begin to think beyond the past in better ways that will help you create the life you really want.

iCan02 - Beyond Positive Thinking
You will discover the secrets to moving beyond positive thinking into a world of infinite possibilities where your other-than-conscious can take over and put your success on autopilot.

iCan03 - Change Your Inner Self Talk – Change Your Life
Journey through this mental exercise that will have you making your positive change in days instead of months. With the right inner talk, powerful action can take place.

iCan04 - Taking the 1st Step to Your – 'I Can' Action
You will learn to transform negative behaviors into positive patterns of improvement. Imagine your life when procrastination leads to motivation and when fear transforms into personal power.

iCan05 - Creating Your 'I Can' – Challenge Breakthroughs
You will learn to plan for success instead of counting on failure. Today is the day you choose to succeed, knowing that the way you do the smallest of things is the way you do the big things.

iCan06 - Living The Dream…Infinite – Possibilities & Opportunities
You will employ your access to an infinite mind. Dr. Porter will teach you the time-tested techniques used by the world's greatest inventors to awaken the genius in your dreams.

Life Mastery

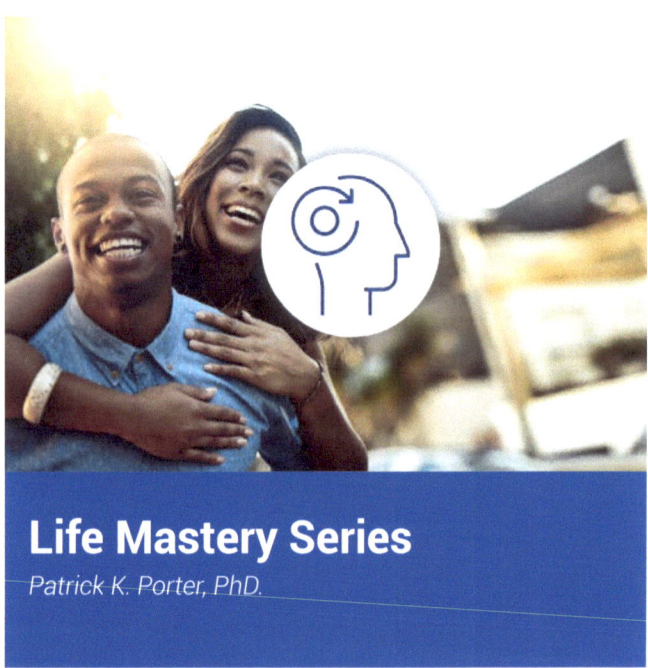

Life Mastery Series
Patrick K. Porter, PhD.

Throughout your life, from parents, teachers, and society, you were taught *what* to think. In this series you are going to discover *how* to think. With this knowledge, you will become a software engineer for your own mind. On the Life-Mastery journey, you will explore limitless ways to achieve personal improvement and success in your life.

LM01 - Operating in Your Optimal Risk Zone
You will learn the mindset of the controlled risk-takers who launched the high-tech industry. You will learn that those thoughts and behaviors can be virtually downloaded into your mind.

LM02 - Ask, Believe & Receive Visualization
You will discover how to be an active participant in the enfoldment of your relationships, wealth, and happiness. Now, without even trying, success will come natural to you.

LM03 - The Secret Power of Self-talk
Learn how to rid your mind of negative thoughts, focusing on positive thoughts, using the same four-step process that has helped thousands of people neutralize fear, anxiety, and worry.

LM04 – Activate the Magnetic Power of Your Dreams
Dreams are a powerful way to communicate with the other-than-conscious mind. You will discover creative ways to use your dreams to visualize solutions to everyday problems.

LM05 – Become a Personal Success Magnet
We all would love to know the secrets of success. In this session, you will tap into your mind's storehouse of thoughts that will act as a magnet, drawing the right people and opportunities to you.

LM06 – Whole Brain Motivation & Unending Drive
You will discover new ways of tapping into the creative right side of your brain, while using the left logical side of the brain to create a timeline for success.

LM07 – Step on The Fast Track to Personal Success
You will explore The Picasso Factor, and find out why it was easy for Gandhi, Einstein, and other masters to put their success on autopilot. You will tap into your own inner genius and be on the fast track to success.

LM08 – Enthusiasm, Focus & Flexibility… Your Keys to Success
YOU will find your own internal success coach, who will take you step-by-step in the direction of your goals. You will make significant progress once you know how to generate the enthusiasm, focus, and flexibility you need on a day-to-day basis.

LM09 – Harness the Power of Change
You will discover why change, the only constant in the universe, can be your most powerful ally. When you harness the power of change, you are tapping into the most potent force in the universe.

LM10 – Awaken Your Senses and Create Your Future
Through sight, sound, touch, smell, and taste, your brain takes in information from the world around you. You will harness your senses to magnetize success to you.

LM11 – Power Phrases for Powerful Actions
Our words have power, so negative words can cause negative effects, and vice versa. You will discover how affirmative words and phrases can create a powerful mental image of a healthy, wealthy, and vibrant new you.

LM12 – Eliminate Negative Thinking and Harness the Power of Optimism
Break through the clutter and activate your optimistic mind. Imagine your new life as you eliminate the negativity and create instantaneous, positive solutions.

LM13 - Transform Procrastination into Total Motivation
This seven-step transformation process will end procrastination, and convert that energy into the usable motivation you'll need to complete tasks, start new projects, and lead a healthy lifestyle.

LM14 – Journey to the Creativity Zone
Creativity is essential to our work performance and is vital in leading a balanced life. Take an inner journey to the place in your mind where ideas abound and solutions are readily available.

Lyme Relief

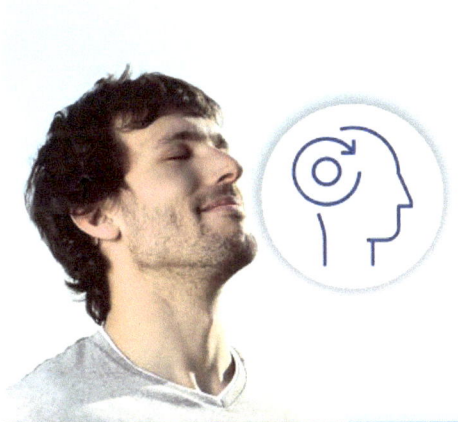

Natural Lyme Relief Breakthrough
Patrick K. Porter, PhD. &
Charmaine Bassett PSC, SC, NMD, DM

Lyme disease is a bacterial illness, transmitted to humans by the bite of deer ticks carrying a bacterium known as Borrelia burgdorferi. Lyme is a systemic issue that can ruin lives. While the medical community continues to make advances, Patrick K Porter, PhD and Charmaine Bassett (PSC, SC, NMD, DM), Chief of Nemenhah Seminaries Services, designed this Natural Lyme Relief Breakthrough series based on Ms. Bassett's 35 years in the health/nutrition field. The series is designed to guide the user through a series of mental exercises to balance brain waves and approach natural healing with a positive attitude, trusting that the power that made the body can heal the body.

IMPORTANT! This series is intended to address habits and lifestyle choices while enhancing spiritual faith and should never be used in place of professional medical or mental health intervention.

LR01 - Deep Relaxation for Lyme Relief
You will train your brain to focus on the natural healing processes of the body, while eliminating the trauma of the experience.

LR02 - Lyme Headache Relief
You will learn the relaxation techniques that will help you eliminate headache pain by turning on the most powerful pharmacy on earth, your human brain.

LR03 - Lyme Joint Pain Relief
As you learn to master the relaxation response, you will discover new ways to train your brain to master pain and live an active life with far more comfort.

LR04 - Supercharge Your Immune System
Through deep relaxation and brainwave entrainment, your symptoms of post Lyme Disease can decrease and your immune system can be super-charged.

LR05 - Rebuilding Your Natural Sleep Response
Stress, worry, and sleepless nights are all common with Lyme. This session will train your brain to return to its natural sleep cycle, allowing you to awaken rested, relaxed, and renewed.

LR06 – Relax and Listen to Your Heart
You will tune into innate intelligence and allow the power that made the body, heal the body. The key is a heart healthy diet, positive thinking, and deep relaxation to recharge the body.

LR07 – Mind/Body Lyme Relief
You will learn mind/body balance, while learning to be assertive, ask for what you need, and build your support team so that you stay on the path to recovery.

Medical

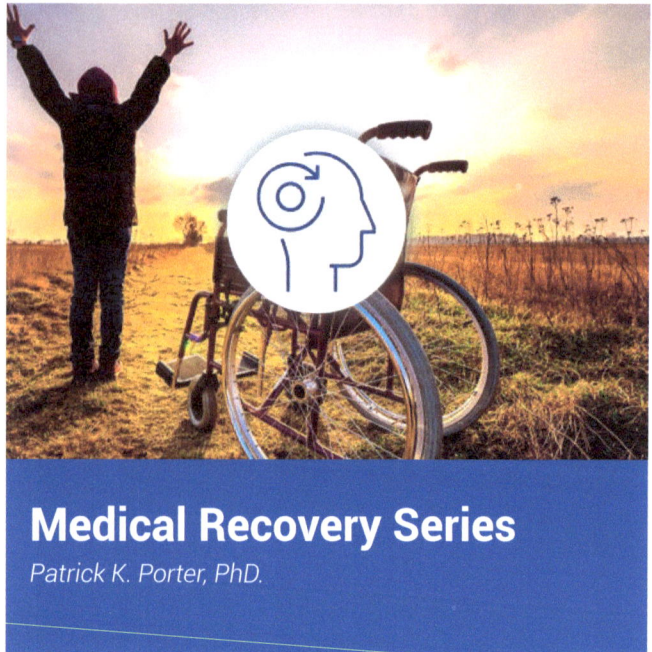

Medical Recovery Series
Patrick K. Porter, PhD.

This series is designed to help you before, during, and after surgical procedures. The initial session begins by showing you how to lower your blood pressure and remain calm. This will benefit you before going in to have a surgical procedure performed. If you are stressed, this may lead to higher blood pressure and your recovery process will take longer. You will learn how to get rid of pre-surgery jitters, and mentally prepare for the procedure. You will be able to relax and remain calm during the procedure. Afterwards, you will be focused on healing while using the tools you learned from these sessions to help you through this time.

MS001 – De-Stress and Lower Blood Pressure
Stress can cause your blood pressure to raise to levels higher than usual. During this session you will learn to achieve the relaxation response and return your blood pressure to a healthy level.

MS02 – Pre-Surgery Calm for Better Healing
You will learn guided relaxation, intense concentration, and focused attention prior to surgery. These techniques can lead to less pain, less medication, and a more rapid recovery.

MS03 – Post-Surgery Stress Relief for a Healthy Mind and Body
Learn a relaxation technique that uses concentration and deep breathing to calm the mind and put your body in the best possible state for repair and healing.

MS04 – Soothing Pain Relief for Rapid Healing
Experiencing some pain post-surgery is expected. You will learn the relaxation response in order to trigger your body into producing its own pain relief.

MS05 – Rid Your Mind of Pre-Surgery Jitters
It is natural to be apprehensive before your surgical procedure. This session will help ease fears and soothe anxiety before surgery.

MS06 – Mentally Prepare for Your Procedure
Relaxing can seem almost impossible before surgery. You will learn how to deal with anxiety, and develop a positive mental attitude, focusing on the success of the procedure.

MS07 – Relax and Heal After Surgery
You will learn how to do quick mental healing sessions throughout the day. You will no longer focus on stress or pain, but begin concentrating on the healing process.

MS08 – Mental Relaxation During a Procedure
With your doctor's approval, you can use this session throughout the procedure to help you relax and focus. This mental relaxation helps decrease stress and can reduce or eliminate discomfort.

MS09 – Staying Relaxed After Your Procedure
You will learn creative ways to relax your mind and body so you sleep deeply, rest completely, and are less impacted by tension and pain.

MS10 – Post-Surgery Visualization for Body Mending
With this session you will discover ways to eliminate insomnia, picturing your body mending after surgery during deep, restful sleep.

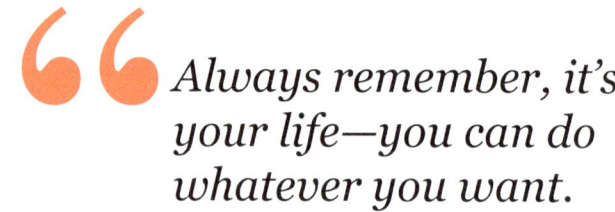

Always remember, it's your life—you can do whatever you want.
~Patrick K Porter PhD

Meditation Switches Off Disease-Causing Genes

Deep relaxation seems to switch off disease-causing genes, according to researchers at Harvard Medical School, while switching on genes that actively protect us from disorders such as high blood pressure to pain to infertility and even rheumatoid arthritis. They attribute these changes to a phenomenon they call the Relaxation Response.

The study compared the genetic profiles of individuals who were long-term practitioners of relaxation methods such as yoga and meditation to a control group of individuals who were not relaxation practitioners.

In the words of lead researcher Dr Herbert Benson, "We found a range of disease fighting genes that were active in the relaxation practitioners but not active in the control group." Interestingly, in as little as two months after the control group began meditating, their genetic profile changed to resemble those of the relaxation practitioners.

Meditation is a term coined to encompass a variety of practices that help you focus your attention and control your thoughts. It is not just a way for us to get in touch with ourselves and calm a busy mind. It appears that, by improving our spiritual and mental health, meditation is also responsible for our genetic health.

The BrainTap audio-sessions found in this catalog are effective tools for creating a relaxed meditative experience, even for those who have never meditated.

The BrainTap headset channels precise frequencies of light and sound and pulsed magnetic fields through the headphones and the glasses directly to the brain, with the intention of creating deep meditative states at the touch of a button. Also, the stimulation from the lights and tones cause the brain to release or step up production of the brain chemicals associated with pleasure, positive mood and memory.

With BrainTap, we can make abnormal brainwave patterns normal, which makes the brain better at self-regulating, creating a positive rippling effect on all cells, tissues, organs, glands and systems of the body.

References:
1. http://www.youramazingbrain.org.uk/brainchanges/stressbrain.htm
2. http://www.meditationcommunity.com/benefits.html
3. http://www.psychologytoday.com/articles/index.php?term=pto-2191.html
5. http://www.newsweek.com/id/141984?from=rss
4. Mind and Body by Priya D. Lal. Published by Gyan Books, 2002

Meditation

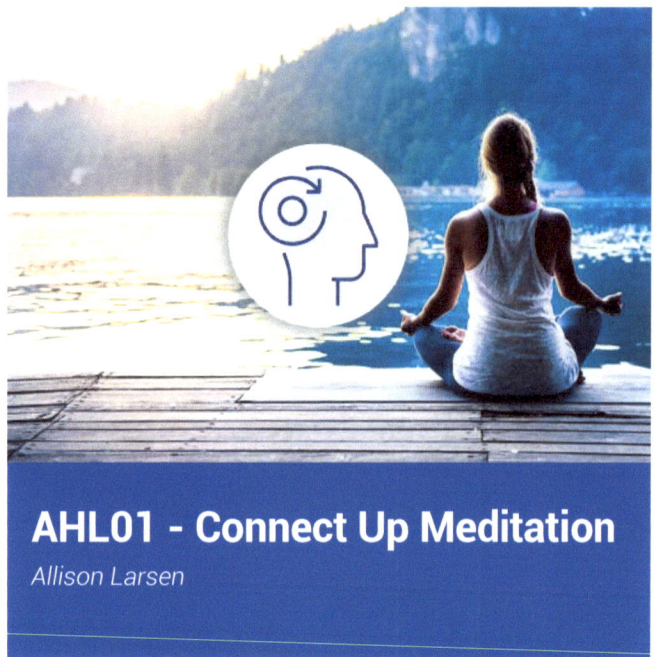

AHL01 - Connect Up Meditation
Allison Larsen

You will release stress and tension throughout your entire body, starting from the crown of your head, moving down to your chest, your stomach, hips, legs, and feet, ending in a calm and relaxed state. You will also release stress and tension from your mind in order to eliminate negativity, worries, or fears.

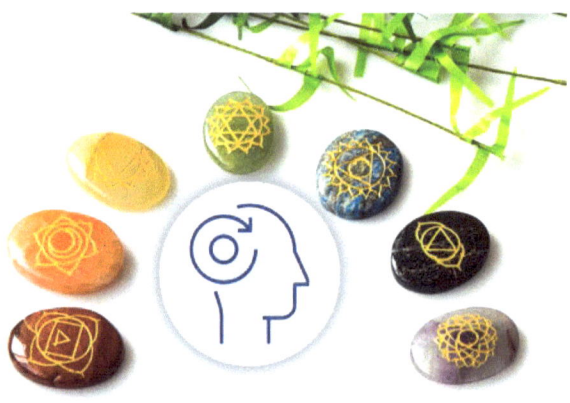

Chakra Meditations
Dr. Donna Perillo

These seven chakras represent something special and unique within your body, and we have all used them at some point in life, either knowingly or unknowingly. You will be able to tap into each chakra with these 10-minute sessions and learn what they are used for, and what should happen when they are balanced. You just need to get comfortable and relaxed, free from any distractions, and allow Dr. Donna Perillo to guide you through each chakra.

DP01 - 1st Chakra - Safety/Security/Survival
This first chakra is known as the root chakra, and begins at the base of the spine. It is associated with the reproductive organs, the immune system, and the color red. Once the root chakra is balanced you will experience unlimited intuition.

DP02 - 2nd Chakra - Feelings/Emotion/Creativity
This chakra is also known as the sacral chakra. It is associated with feeling accepted or rejected, or a sense of belonging. The color associated with this chakra is orange. After this meditation you may experience childlike feelings.

DP03 - 3rd Chakra - Power Zone
This chakra is known as the solar plexuss. It is associated with your relationships to others in the world and the color yellow. You will be able to make major decisions that best benefit yourself and others.

DP04 - 4th Chakra - Heart/Love
This chakra is known as the heart chakra. When this chakra is balanced, you feel a sense of unconditional love and connectedness to humanity. It is associated with the color green. You will experience a sense of peace, regardless of what is going on around you.

DP05 - 5th Chakra - Communication
This chakra is known as the throat chakra. When it is balanced you are able to separate emotional and physical functions of the body from each other. It gives off the color blue. You will be able to speak and communicate accurately and effectively.

DP06 - 6th Chakra - Intuition/Perception
This chakra is known as the third eye. It controls the incoming and outgoing messages of the brain, and also taps into paranormal activity. It radiates a red-blue color similar to violet. You will be able to merge your conscious and unconscious and experience your higher self.

DP07 - 7th Chakra - Spirituality/Perception
This chakra is known as the head heart center and is located at the top of the head. It is associated with the color violet. You will experience self-realization.

DP08 - Body Scan - Finding the Stress in Your Body
The purpose of the body scan is to relax you and focus on each area of your body. You will be able to realize which chakras need the most work. If you feel any tension or pain you will able to release it throughout your entire body.

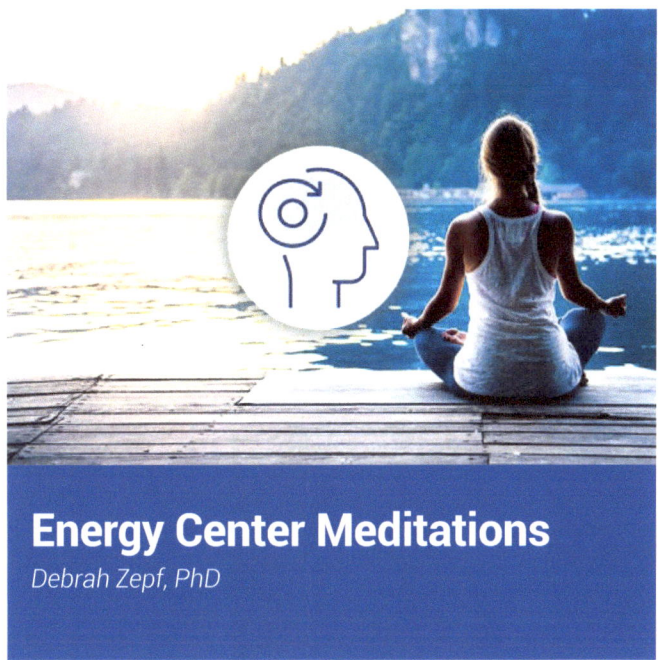

Energy Center Meditations
Debrah Zepf, PhD

During these 15-17 minute sessions, you will balance your energy centers by learning what each of the seven chakras is used for, as well as the some of the advantages and disadvantages of each. All you need to do is relax and allow Dr. Debrah Zepf to guide you through each energy center.

ECM01 - 1st Energy Center Meditation Root Chakra
Life force energy is our connection to earth and the material world. We call it the root chakra because it gives us stability in life and initiates new beginnings. This session will help stabilize the foundation of your body's energy.

ECM02 - 2nd Energy Center Meditation Sacral Chakra
Emotions, addictions, and violence are all associated with this chakra. The session for this second energy center is very unique and it was created to bring peace and balance, and to open us to simple healing pleasures.

ECM03 - 3rd Energy Center Meditation Solar Plexus Chakra
The solar plexus chakra is where we release all that is not for our highest good so we can receive abundance. This session assists with clearing the chakra and is used mainly for anxiety, lowering cholesterol, and blood pressure.

ECM04 - 4th Energy Center Meditation Heart Chakra
This session facilitates the oneness to restore faith and find love. The heart chakra is associated with the respiratory system and is used for fevers, emotional, and heart challenges, but it also calms and harmonizes your mind and body.

ECM05 - 5th Energy Center Meditation Throat Chakra
Activate the healing within so that you can have integrity and peace and share the wisdom of living our truth. The throat chakra may be associated with problems in the thyroid, parathyroid, teeth, and lymphatic challenges, however it is known to help with allergies, digestion, injuries, and asthma.

ECM06 - 6th Energy Center Meditation Third Eye Brow Chakra
This meditation helps balance the lower and higher selves so we can trust the inner self. It helps with balancing intellectual, emotional, and physical properties and awakening intuition.

ECM07 - 7th Energy Center Meditation Crown Chakra
This meditation will ground you, inspire you and guide you to the connect as one with the Divine. On the physical level, it can help alleviate sinusitis and it works wonders for insomnia and mild headaches.

ECM08 - 8th Energy Center Meditation Whole Body Bliss
This meditation guides you through the seven energy centers and helps you attain whole body balance. Not only does it help with universal oneness, it gives the body tools to help with the healing process on all levels.

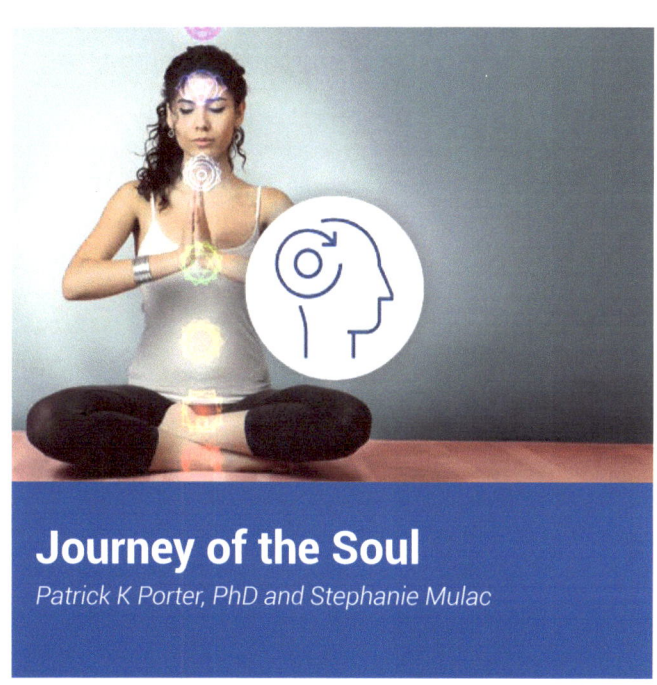

Journey of the Soul
Patrick K Porter, PhD and Stephanie Mulac

This series is designed to help you journey into your soul on different levels. There are sessions dealing with health, wealth, relationships, career moves, personal goals, among other topics. You will learn to commit to your journey in this first session, and realize that you have the power to be great, no matter what you have been led to believe. You will tap into this power and learn to use it throughout this journey of the soul guided by Dr. Patrick Porter.

JOS01 - Committing to Your Journey of the Soul
You may believe you are incapable of achieving your goals. You will acknowledge that you are greater than what you've been led to believe, and allow the skills and abilities of your soul to create everything you desire.

JOS02 - Health and Wellbeing on Your Journey
Health is very important to your wellbeing. During this session you will learn to become drawn to fresh, vibrant foods, and repelled by junk foods.

JOS03 - Wealth and Finance on Your Journey
Often times we set goals, but never accomplish them. During this session you will learn to do whatever it is you wish to do with purpose and passion.

JOS04 - Relationships on Your Journey
You will realize that we live in a relationship with all things. You will start by resolving any inner conflict you have. Then you will learn to build true relationships, no matter who they are with.

JOS05 - Lifestyle Transformation on Your Journey
You will focus on changes that you've always wanted to make but never did. You will learn to do things on your own terms.

JOS06 - Personal Growth on Your Journey
Negative emotions can keep you from pursuing your passion. You will begin to release the fear and frustration preventing you from pursuing your soul's passion.

JOS07 - Career Moves on Your Journey
You will learn to attract someone who possesses the skills and abilities you wish to have. You will build these skills one day at a time in order to become successful.

JOS08 - Inner-State on Your Journey
You will reconnect with mother earth and come to understand the resources you have within yourself and the world. You will ensure your presence on earth is remembered as one of caring for the environment.

JOS09 - Spirituality on Your Journey
Many find spirituality to be complex. You will begin to understand the world around you and your true self. You will then be able to connect with spirituality.

JOS10 - You Have the Power to Change the World
We all have wanted to change something within the world at some point. You will learn to rise above your current situation and realize you can be the change you want to see in the world.

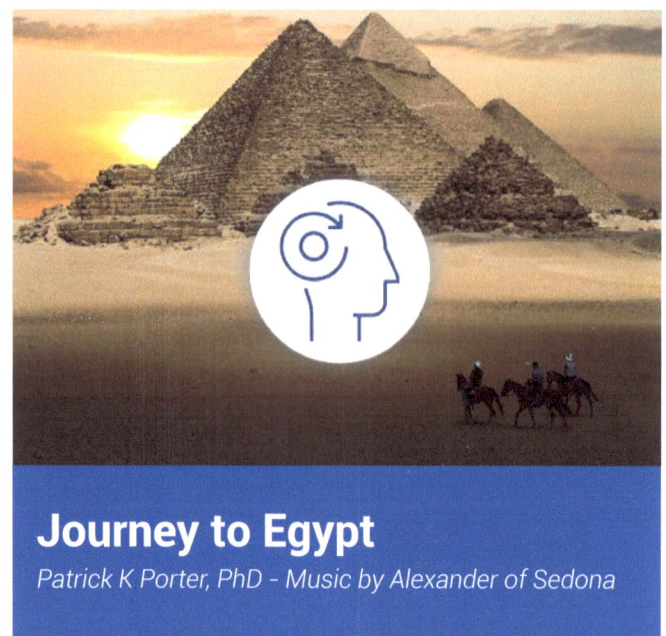

Journey to Egypt
Patrick K Porter, PhD - Music by Alexander of Sedona

During this 42-minute session, you will release any disbeliefs of your ability to travel through space and time. You will allow your mind to drift into times of pre-recorded history. You will imagine yourself lying in the sand along the river Nile as your mind journeys through Egypt.

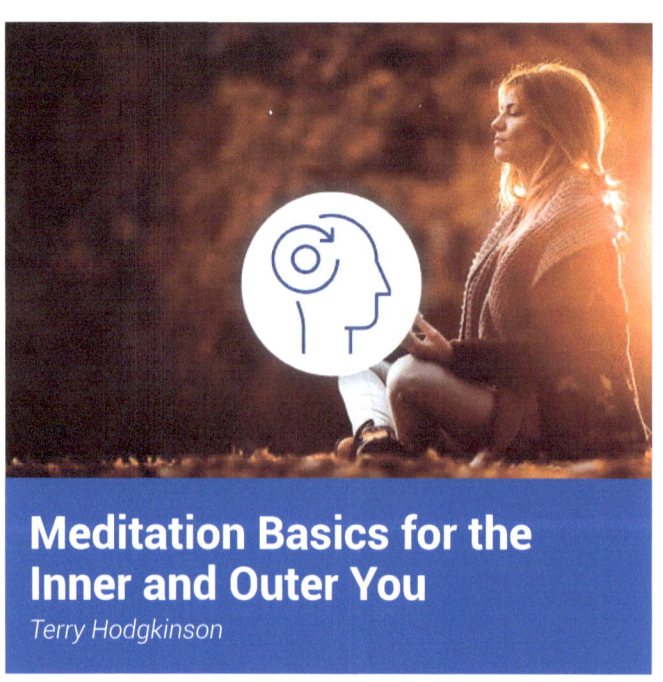

Meditation Basics for the Inner and Outer You
Terry Hodgkinson

Terry Hodgkinson is a meditation master instructor who has experienced the power of the mind through meditation. He designed this series to guide you through these meditations for four weeks. He will cover many aspects of meditation and share some of his experiences throughout.

MBIOY01 - Week 1 Day 1 - How to Start Meditation
In this first meditation session, you will learn the basics of body posture and proper breathing. Once you have the basics down you will reap better results in your meditation practice.

MBIOY02 - Week 1 Day 2 - Your Amazing Mind Meditation
You will penetrate deeper into the ramification of the mind. You will learn how to properly space out your breathing cycles, inhaling through the nose and exhaling through the mouth.

MBIOY03 - Week 1 Day 3 - How the Brain Works Meditation
Our brains are chemical factories that release chemical messengers, which affect our mind and body constantly. If we understand how the brain works, then we can understand how to work the brain.

MBIOY04 - Week 1 Day 4 - The Power of Visualization Meditation
The simple act of using your imagination can make a difference in assisting your brain to bring you the results you desire. You will learn some of the health benefits that conscious aware breath meditation can bring.

MBIOY05 - Week 1 Day 5 - Shifting Gears Meditation
Have you ever felt sad, disappointed, or unhappy, and wished you didn't? You will learn an easy process that will help your mind shift gears, and realize it's much easier than you think.

MBIOY06 - Week 1 Day 6 - Let the Universe Breathe You Meditation
Being able to cherish and look forward to your daily time of meditation practice is vital to your health and happiness. You will put the time you spend on yourself into proper perspective and sync with the universe.

MBIOY07 - Week 1 Day 7 - Five Visuals for Relaxation Meditation
You will be guided through five easy visualizations that will help you obtain inner calm and relaxation. You will establish a continuation of inner calm and relaxation along your life journey.

MBIOY08 - Week 2 Day 8 - Hakuins Butter Egg Meditation
Zen master Hakuin Ekaku used this meditation to revive himself when he became ill. Hakuyu the hermit taught Hakuin this Butter Egg Visualization meditation so he could bring his body back into balance and heal.

MBIOY09 - Week 2 Day 9 - Opening Your Heart
Open your heart and let go of negative thoughts or feelings. You will begin to use your heart qualities, such as joy, compassion, and love, in areas of your life that may lack enjoyment.

MBIOY10 - Week 2 Day 10 - A Ray of Sunshine
You will see that opportunities exist each day from the moment you open your eyes until you close them again to sleep at night. When your mind is right, you will be able to see and appreciate more.

MBIOY11 - Week 2 Day 11 - Enhancing Your Senses
It's amazing how much we filter out of our consciousness due to everyday routines. These exercises will enhance your sensory acuity to become aware of and appreciate the simple things in life.

MBIOY12 - Week 2 Day 12 - Pebbles in the Pond
You will listen to three interesting visualizations, the last one taking you to a pond where pebbles are thrown to create waves, just like the waves you create in your life from the thoughts you think.

MBIOY13 - Week 2 Day 13 - Cultivate Your Inner Sanctuary
You will discover your inner sanctuary. Once you know how to cultivate inner peace you will be amazed at what you can achieve.

MBIOY14 - Week 2 Day 14 - Journey Inside the Body
You will be taken on a journey inside your body. You will get to see, understand, and appreciate what your lungs and heart do for you and how your body works harmoniously.

MBIOY15 - Week 3 Day 15 - Rain Flowers and Stars
Whether you place your thoughts on negativity or positivity, that feeling will only grow stronger. You will learn to focus your attention on joy, and realize it can be found in every aspect of life.

MBIOY16 - Week 3 Day16 - Gratitude
Often times it's the simple things in life that bring us joy, but are taken for granted. You will spend more time meditating on what you have to be thankful for.

MBIOY17 - Week 3 Day 17 - Happy Birthday Brain
You will learn that every day you can experience a birthday, and celebrate the fact that your brain is capable of fresh new thoughts, invigorating ideas, and stimulating beliefs.

MBIOY18 - Week 3 Day 18 - Journey into Awareness
Examples of hot air balloons, fish, and getting your black belt show why awareness is the key to understanding yourself, others, and our journey called life.

MBIOY19 - Week 3 Day 19 - Cleaning Memories in Mind
You will be lead through the hallway of memories in your mind and shown a way to reorganize those memories so the good ones are in the forefront, while the negative ones are further back.

MBIOY20 - Week 3 Day 20 - Walk Through Beliefs
Just because your beliefs are a particular way right now, doesn't mean they will always remain that way. When you are open to discovering the truth, you will see how often past beliefs have changed.

MBIOY21 - Week 3 Day 21 - The Sun Within Any Storm
No storm lasts forever. You will learn to relax when life gets challenging so you can watch the storm go by. The sun will soon come out again.

MBIOY22 - Week 4 Day 22 - Going With The Flow
You will learn to let go and go with the flow. You will realize that your perception can be altered to recognize and appreciate everyday life situations.

MBIOY23 - Week 4 Day 23 - A Greater Freedom
You will be able to connect with a greater freedom that resides within you. Most people look for this peace on the outside, when they should really look within.

MBIOY24 - Week 4 Day 24 - A Peaceful World
We all know danger and violence exist, but too many people focus on only that. You will be guided through a world of peace. The more you visualize a peaceful world, the more joyful it will be.

MBIOY25 - Week 4 Day 25 Intelligent Beliefs
When you don't give a goal any effort, it's usually because you believe that you cannot succeed. You will understand how powerful your beliefs are and learn to make positive changes.

MBIOY26 - Week04 Day26 Feeling Connected
We may not see the connection between things, but that does not mean it's not there. You will explore the deeper connection between your mind, heart, and all living things.

MBIOY27 - Week 4 Day 27 - Journey to Dharamsala
You will journey to Dharamsala, India. You will listen to the same music performed by monks at the monastery.

MBIOY28 - Week 4 Day 28 - The Sweat Lodge Ceremony
Sweat Lodge Ceremonies are to cleanse physically, mentally, emotionally, and spiritually. You will hear segments of songs, chants, and music specifically used for this ceremony performed by Dennis Hawk.

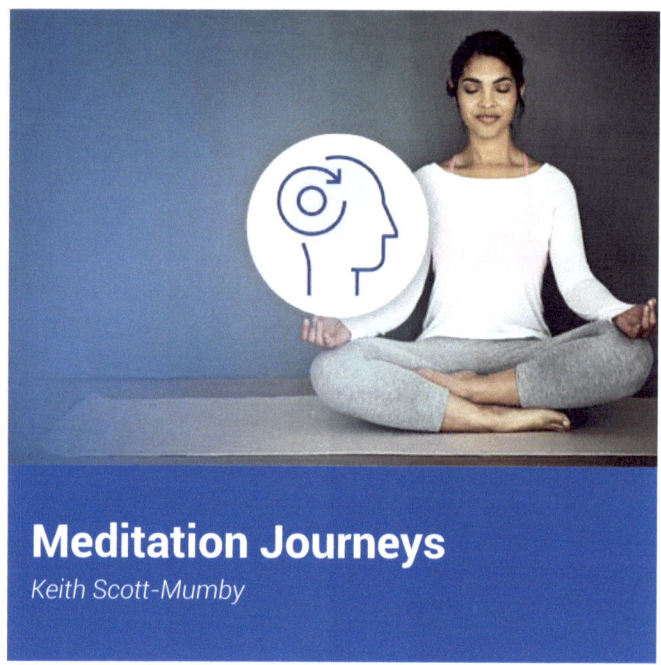

Meditation Journeys
Keith Scott-Mumby

Keith Scott-Mumby will guide your mind through travels to several different places you didn't realize you could go. You will also embark on journeys of forgiveness, goodness, gratitude, and love. You will be amazed at the different places you can go when you learn to relax your mind and body. These electronically enhanced journeys will allow you to delve deep within and focus on what is meaningful, positive, and good.

Avalon
You will allow your mind to travel to Avalon where King Arthur came from. This place doesn't have to be real, you can simply allow yourself to travel to another dimension.

Forgiveness Process
Many people have a fixed idea that forgiving someone excuses them for what they did. With this meditation you will learn the power of forgiveness. You will learn to humble yourself and let go.

Goodness Meditation
What if you were remembered by your worst act? What impression would you leave? In this session you will rewrite the past and focus on what is moral and good.

Gratitude Process
Expressing gratitude releases the hold pain may have on our hearts and minds. You will be encouraged to list five things you are grateful for daily. You will focus on positivity to change your perspective on life.

Journey to Atlantis
You will journey to the famous lost world known as Atlantis, a peaceful location where you can escape the stress most

of us encounter in today's world. You will be able to take something positive away from this journey once it's over.

Love Process
Love is not something we give, we get, or we do. It is what we are. You will learn embrace this truth during and take a journey on the pursuit of love and happiness.

Tour of the Universe
You will shut out the world and focus within. You will journey around the universe, and open up your mind and soul to travels beyond the body.

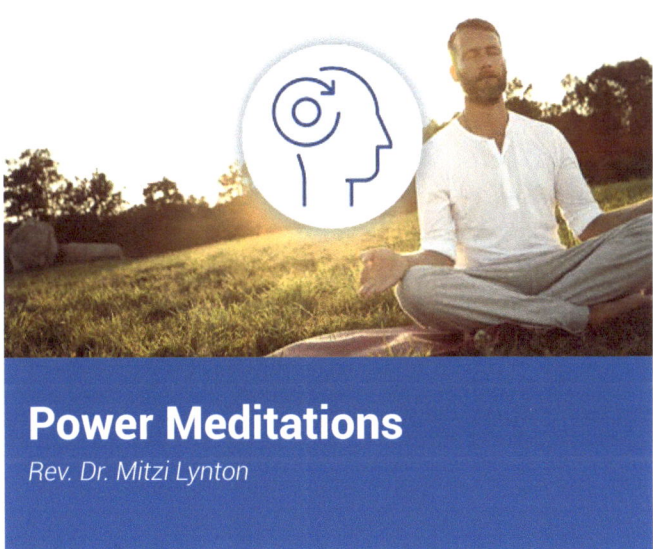

Power Meditations
Rev. Dr. Mitzi Lynton

You will remove any unwanted stress and tension from your body and learn to relax. You will imagine yourself becoming one with nature in several sessions and enjoy the elements of nature around you. You will also gain confidence in yourself and release any fears you may have. This inspiring series will leave you with a feeling of relaxation and rejuvenation.

CRVSR10 - Mitzi
You will bring up unwanted stressful emotions in order to allow your mind to develop a spontaneous relaxation response. You will be able to remain more relaxed in stressful situations that would normally cause you to be uptight.

CVRSR01 - Mitzi
You will tap into the library of your mind. It will be your place to remove all stress from your mind and body's awareness. You will be able to journey to this quiet, serene place whenever you're experiencing stress.

CVRSR02 - Mitzi
We all get caught up with the stress and strain of everyday life. This session will take you on a mental vacation. You will awaken feeling refreshed, revitalized, and renewed.

MLY01 - Discover Your Power Word
You will release any discomfort about being in the moment. You will listen to the sounds of nature, the wind blowing and the water running over the rocks. You will feel refreshed and at peace.

MLY02 - Pot of Gold Abundance Visualization
You will imagine walking along a path in the forest on a nice, sunny day. Your body will be at peace and at ease. All you need to do is relax and enjoy this mental walk.

MLY03 - Releasing Fear
Fear may be blocking you from pursuing what it is you truly desire. You will realize that there is nothing to fear and you are safe. You will feel relaxed and at complete peace.

MLY04 - Your Time to Shine
You will realize that today is your time to shine. You will accomplish what it is you intended to do with a smile on your face. You will feel empowered knowing you put your best foot forward.

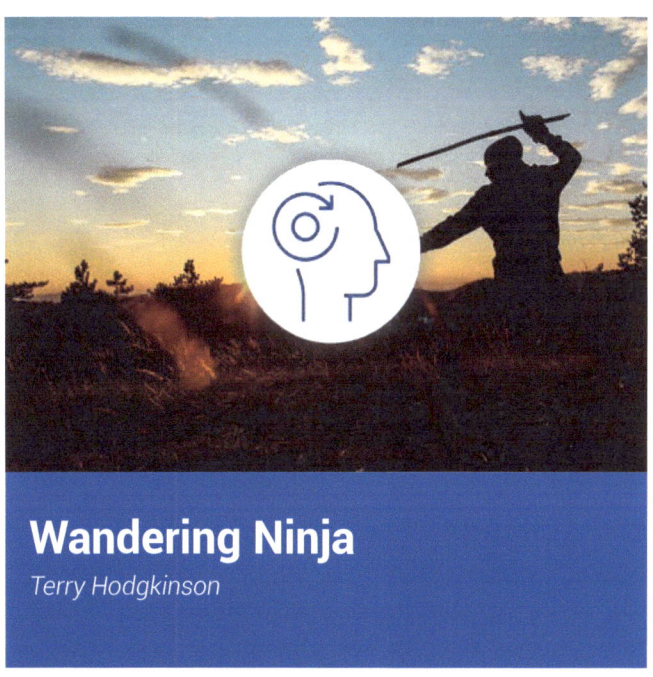

Wandering Ninja
Terry Hodgkinson

This series is based on the book, *Memoirs of a Wandering Ninja,* by Terry Hodgkinson, an exceptional martial arts instructor, meditation teacher and spiritual retreat leader. You will take a virtual journey with a martial arts expert and meditation master to some of the most remote yet spiritually awakened destinations on earth.

These memoirs are steeped in essential timeless wisdom gathered from not only spiritual sages but also from lessons taught by ancient micro-cultures hidden in such faraway places as the forests and jungles of China, Thailand, Vietnam, Cambodia and India. These principles have withstood the test of time from martial arts masters and sages. However, you do not need to be a martial arts master or student to benefit by traveling this path. Rather, you need only be a seeker of spiritual truth. Join Terry in his travels as he openly shares his insights that put you in harmony with the natural laws of the universe, and will awaken your spiritual body.

WN01 - Panther Stillness Meditation
Panthers have the ability to sit still for long periods of time, while absorbing everything in their surroundings. You will gain this ability to remain calm in any environment or situation, with pure awareness.

WN02 - Eagle Vision Meditation
Being too close and attached to something can obstruct your vision of that object, especially if you're emotionally invested. You will gain a bird's eye view by distancing yourself and gaining a different perspective on the situation.

WN03 - Transforming Water Meditation
Water can transform into a solid (ice), liquid (water), or a gas (water vapor), and still be H2O. YOu will learn to transform your perception of situations and realize the grass is not always greener on the other side.

WN04 - Immovable Mountain Meditation
Mountains represent strength and stability. You will journey to a peaceful mountain, where you will envision yourself handling situations from an empowering state of mind.

WN05 - Sunrises Energize
Sunrise represents the start of a new day. You will tap into the renewing energy that occurs with each new day and learn to make the best of it.

WN06 - Summoning Mountain Meditation
This session is similar to that of the immovable mountain meditation, however, you will summon your strongest resources in order to achieve your desired outcome for any situation.

WN07 - Animal Spirit
The monks reasoned that, if you learn to possess the qualities of certain animals, you will learn their superior capabilities of self-defense. You will tap into your animal spirit and develop new skills you never knew you had.

WN08 - Grateful Harvest Meditation
The power of gratitude should never be underestimated. You will learn to give and receive gratitude. When you experience gratitude you will feel a sense of peace.

Menopause

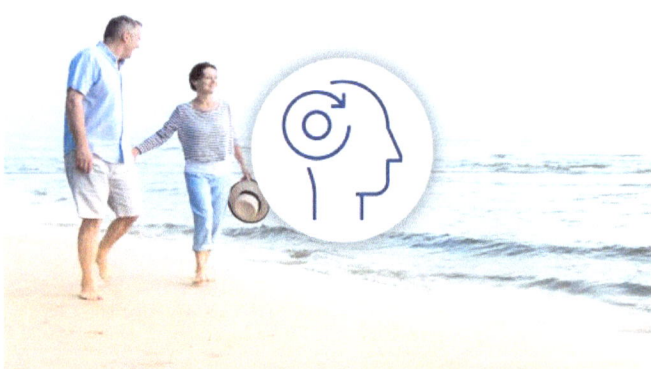

Mind-Over-Menopause
Patrick K. Porter, Ph.D.

For many women, mid-life can be a time of uncertainty and loss. For some, the loss of fertility and the perceived loss of youth can cause depression and anxiety. At the same time, the body's response to the decrease in hormones can create any number of symptoms—hot flashes, night sweats, weight gain, itchy skin, mood swings, lost libido, headaches, and irregular cycles are just of few of the menopausal challenges women face. In the midst of all these changes, relationships can suffer as loved ones start to ask, "What happened to the caring, loving woman we once knew?" Now you can reclaim that woman, along with all the strength, confidence, and wisdom you gained in the first half of your life. This series takes you way beyond mind over matter, it's mind over menopause!

IMPORTANT! This series is intended to address habits and lifestyle choices while enhancing spiritual faith and should never be used in place of professional medical or mental health intervention.

MM01 - Balance Your Mood, Balance Your Life
You will learn to relax, balance your mood, and utilize your positive mental energy. You will stop focusing on what you've lost, and discover all that you've gained!

MM02 - Creating Harmony With the Cycles of Life
This session will show you how to use your mind to activate the powerful, calming effects produced by your brain chemistry, making the emotional ups and downs of menopause a distant memory.

MM03 - Mental Skills to Help You Master Menopause
You will start planning your life from a new perspective. You will learn to view menopause as a rite of passage that gives you confidence and inner worth.

MM04 - Relax and Control Night Sweats and Hot Flashes
You will learn to use relaxation therapy as a natural remedy for hot flashes. You will discover that you can master the cooling effects of your mind and let it cool your body your body well.

MM05 - Eliminate Brain Fog and Sharpen Your Memory
During menopause, many women describe a lack of focus and concentration, commonly known as brain fog. This session will help end this fog, improve your memory, and end confusion and overwhelm.

MM06 - Coping With Emotional Changes During Menopause
You may feel your emotions are getting the best of you. In this session, you will build healthy coping mechanisms for conquering mood swings, overcoming anxiety, and regaining your libido.

MM07 - Get Connected in Times of Uncertainty
Many menopausal women describe feeling disconnected from their bodies. During this session you will discover a new sense of connectedness and purpose, and your "woman's intuition" will be back in full swing!

MM08 - Eliminate Fatigue and Boost Your Energy
Menopause can cause feelings of fatigue and low energy. This session will show you how to own your personal space, develop an emotional drive to make your well-being a top priority and feel your fatigue melt away.

MM09 - Mastering the Physical Changes of Menopause
Gastrointestinal distress, nausea, and headaches are common changes associated with menopause. During this session you will put a plan into action for controlling these issues by thinking and engaging the internal pharmacy within your brain.

MM10 - Tips for Quick Menopausal Relief
You will create a new, healthier lifestyle that includes cutting back on caffeine, alcohol, and spicy foods the easy way. You can sit back, relax, and let these tips for reducing stress and clearing your head take you away.

MM11 - Making Peace With Your Body
Menopause can come with unusual symptoms, such as an annoying buzzing in your head, electric shock sensations, dry mouth, dry eyes, dizziness, or lightheadedness. This session is like Tai Chi for the mind, where you will discover new ways to handle these symptoms.

MM12 - Pain Control and Menopause
You may experience sore joints and muscles, cramps, or headaches with menopause. You will learn a simple, yet powerful process to put your pain at bay, however, any undiagnosed pain should be reported to your medical professional.

MM13 - Three Easy Steps To Regaining Balance
Many women experience irregular cycles and mood swings while transitioning into menopause. With this session, you will learn the three simple steps needed to regain balance in your life, no matter the circumstances.

Musical Journeys

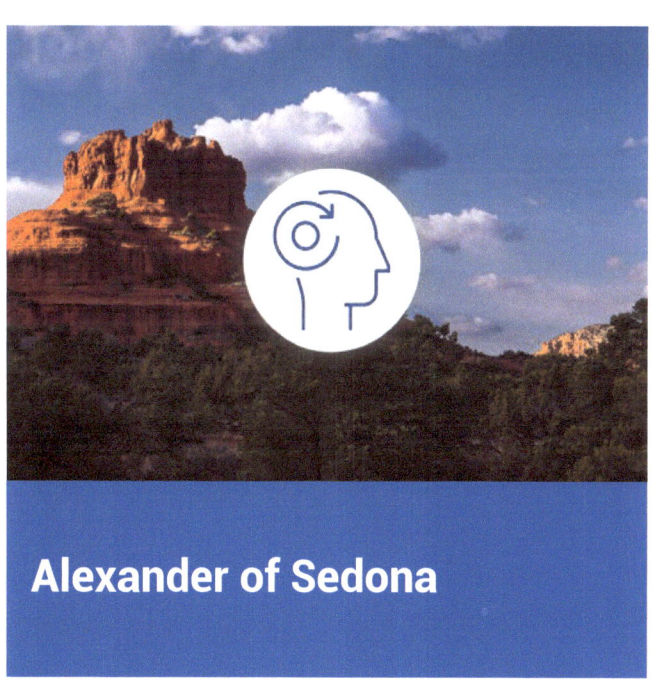

Alexander of Sedona

You will journey to a place of calmness and serenity. Allow the wind dance and waters of life sessions to take you to a tranquil place in your mind where you can be at peace.

Alex01 - Wind Dance
With this session you will experience calming, peaceful music that will allow you to relax.

Alex02 - Waters of Life
You will experience peace and tranquility as you listen to the waters of life.

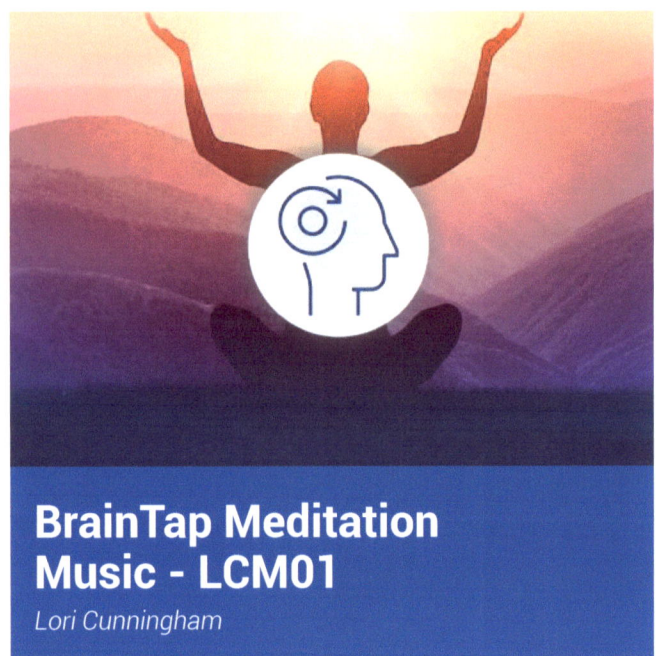

BrainTap Meditation Music - LCM01
Lori Cunningham

This session is a 20-minute theta training set to beautiful, relaxing, soothing love song played by Lori Cunningham. All you need to do is relax and enjoy this 20 minute melody.

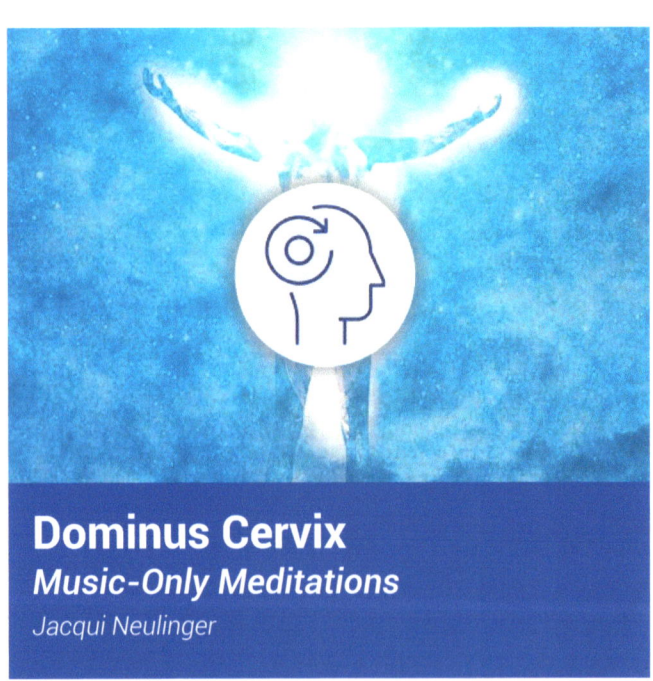

Dominus Cervix
Music-Only Meditations
Jacqui Neulinger

Dominus Cervix is a latin term that refers to the original light port, located at the nape of the neck that was believed to be where the soul enters the body. It is also an intelligent energy. The energies join together to create a network that cleanses your body, your home, and your environment. The music that you will experience in this series will start the process of optimal cleansing, healing, and growth on a spiritual, emotional, physical, and mental level.

SGSD01 - Cleansing of House and Environment
Cleansing is very important. With this 4-minute session you will feel the energy that initiates cleansing of your home and environment. There is no better feeling than that of a refreshing home.

SGSD02 - Cleansing and Healing of the Body and Soul
During this 4-minute session you will feel the energy associated with healing your body and soul. You will experience feelings of happiness and positivity, while stimulating your mental and spiritual growth.

SGSD03 - Geometric Meditation MindFit LBB
Helps to harnesses the power of sacred geometry and to create an experience of deep inner purification and activation of the light body. You will experience an opportunity of profoundly deep physical, mental, emotional, and spiritual transformation.

SGSD04 - Cleansing of House and Environment - Intense
This 4-minute session is an intensified version of cleansing your house and environment. You will experience stronger energy released into your home, that will provide you a more calm, peaceful, and relaxed environment.

SGSD05 - Full Mix
This session is a 42 minute full mix of the different meditations in this series, including cleansing of house and environment, cleansing and healing of the body and soul, and geometric meditation. This session will release energy to help cleanse you on every level.

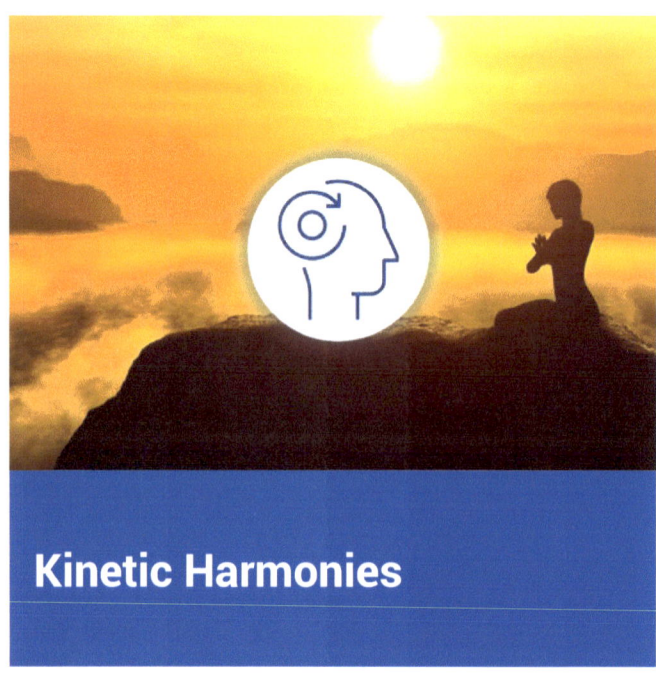

Kinetic Harmonies

During this series you will listen to relaxing, soothing music that will help balance your chakras, help release depression, find divine peace, and tap into the water of life. So sit back and enjoy these calming sessions.

VAL01 - Chakra Journey (30 Mins)
Throughout this journey you will listen to relaxing sounds that will allow you to balance your chakras.

VAL02 - Depression Release (20 Mins)
This session will help you relax and release any depression you may be experiencing.

VAL03 - Divine Peace (30 Mins)
You will experience divine peace while listening to this relaxing session.

VAL04 - Water of Life (7 Mins)
This calming, soothing music will help you tap into the water of life.

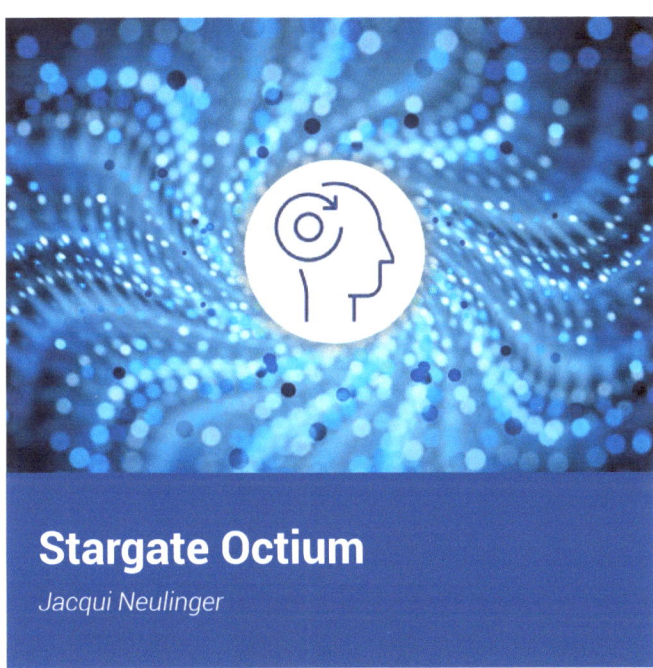

Stargate Octium
Jacqui Neulinger

In these sessions you will experience calming music that will release positive energy into the atmosphere, and allow transformation on a spiritual, emotional, mental, and physical level. You can relax and enjoy these brief sessions, and also enjoy a complete mix of all the sessions.

SGSO01-3 Stargate Octium Part 1-3
You will experience soothing music that will release positive, calming energy into the atmosphere.

SGSO04 - Stargate Complete Mix
This session is a complete mix of sessions 1-3.

Nutrition

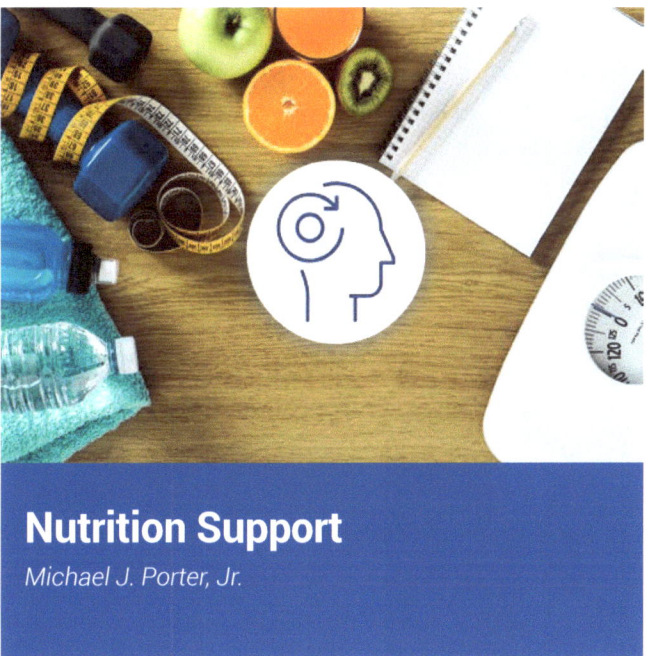

Nutrition Support
Michael J. Porter, Jr.

Nutrition plays a major role in your health. Learning the proper foods to eat and what not to eat will help you keep your body in balance. During this series you will learn things about your body you may not have known, such as how to oxygenate your body and detoxify your body. You will learn how to monitor your sugar intake, how much fiber to include in your diet, as well as protein. If you are struggling with how to properly lose weight, maintain healthy, and balance your body, this is the series for you. These 21 sessions will cover everything you need to know and more about nutrition.

IMPORTANT! This series is intended to promote healthy eating strategies and should never be used in place of professional medical intervention.

NS01 – Understanding the Body: The Acid Alkaline Balance
Many people do not understand their bodies. This session is designed to reinforce the steps that you need to take to keep your body in balance.

NS02 – Oxygenating the Body: The Lymphatic System
The lymphatic system helps your body eliminate waste products from the cells. This session will stimulate your mind and body to rejuvenate itself from the inside out.

NS03 – Detoxifying the Body
Faulty elimination causes the body to build up waste. This session will show you how to get your body back on track.

NS04 – Food and Body Chemistry
It's not what you eat, but the balance of what you eat, and the hormonal response created that is important. Your mind will

be stimulated to eat the right food, in the right amount, at the right time.

NS05 – The Importance of Protein and Weight Loss
Trying to lose weight without protein can be difficult. This session will help increase your protein intake and keep you healthy. You will learn the true importance of these structural building blocks of the human system.

NS06 – Sugar Awareness
Sugar and its many substitutes have become a part of most foods today and are hardly noticed. You will learn how to naturally become aware of the hidden sugars in the foods you eat.

NS07 – The Importance of a High Fiber Diet
It can be hard to sustain optimum health without fiber. In this session, you will learn which foods contain the fiber you need to help you improve your health and accelerate weight loss.

NS08 – Enzymes and Minerals
The human body needs certain enzymes and minerals to sustain vitality. You will learn what to avoid to keep the enzymes in your body from being destroyed, and you will no longer desire foods that are not good for your body.

NS09 – Reactive Foods and Weight Loss
You will understand how reactive foods impede the entire process of weight loss and why certain foods make you feel a certain way.

NS10 – Changing Belief Systems: Emotions and Health
You will learn about the essential nutrients that preserve critical brain functions during moments of stress, and be able to properly handle these emotions.

NS11 – Essential Fatty Acids
Contrary to what most people believe, there are good fats and bad fats. You will learn about the foods that contain EFAs (good fats), so you can begin to incorporate them into your nutritional diet.

NS12 – Reversing the Aging Process
You will learn which foods to eat to keep your body oxygenated, helping you live a longer and healthier life for years to come.

NS13 – Understanding the Body's Metabolism
The chemical process inside your body that keeps you alive is known as your metabolism. You will learn how to naturally maximize your metabolism through proper diet and exercise.

NS14 – Breaking Through Plateaus
There comes a point in your weight loss journey, known as the "plateau", effect where you will find it difficult to lose additional weight. You will learn effective exercise tips for breaking through these plateaus.

NS15 – Sample Meals That Will Keep You Naturally Thin
Binge eating and going through long periods without any food slows down your metabolism, and decreases your blood sugar levels. You will learn the correct proportions of carbohydrates, proteins, and EFAs that should be included in your diet.

NS16 – How Stress Affects Weight Loss
Stress is an inevitable part of our lives. In this session, you will learn why adrenaline and cortisol affect your ability to lose weight and how to make the necessary changes.

NS17 – Understanding Neurotransmitters and Hormones
Knowing what to eat, when to eat it, and how much to eat is controlled by the region of your brain called the "hypothalamus." During this session, you will learn the difference between neurotransmitters and hormones that affect your ability to eliminate excess weight.

NS18 – How GLA and CLA Affect Weight Loss
Similar to EFAs, GLA and CLA are considered to be "good" fats that are necessary for improving and maintaining your health. You will gain a better understanding about GLA and CLA, and the impact it has on your ability to lose weight.

NS19 – Recognizing Thyroid Problems
You will learn the symptoms to look out for in a sluggish thyroid. You will also learn the critical functions and substances that affect it in order to recognize when there is a problem.

NS20 – The Importance of Water
Your body will not run efficiently when it is dehydrated. In this session, you will learn why drinking water instead of soda, coffee, and sugary juice drinks is much better for you.

NS21 – Exercise and Weight Loss
When it comes to weight loss, exercise is the foundation that will help create the body and health you deserve. During this session, you will learn the life-changing benefits that exercise can offer you.

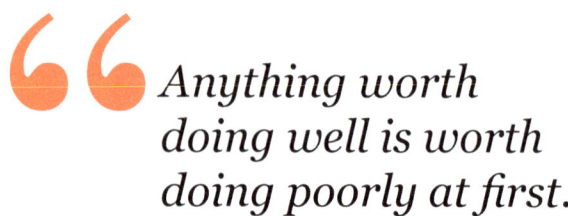

"Anything worth doing well is worth doing poorly at first.
~Patrick K Porter PhD

Why Your Brain is the Best Pharmacy

Do we really have the power in our own minds to create changes in our bodies? That answer is a resounding yes! It's called the placebo effect, and it's many times proven more effective than the drug it's being tested against.

For example, a study on the effectiveness of St. John's Wort versus Zoloft found that both treatments eased symptoms in patients at about the same rate; however, a placebo beat both by more than 8 percent! Why? Because the brain's job is to solve problems. The expectation that something will work is, in many cases, enough to trigger the brain to solve the problem on its own. The placebo effect works because your body has its own natural pharmacy, and it's controlled by the brain.

Neurotransmitters — the Brain's Natural Pharmacy

Neurotransmitters travel a designated path in the brain and affect behavior and emotions. There are two types of neurotransmitters—**excitatory** and **inhibitory.**

Inhibitory neurotransmitters balance mood, but they are depleted quickly when the excitatory neurotransmitters are overactive. When we're in an overly stressed state or thinking negatively, the excitatory neurotransmitters override those that keep our mood balanced—which can quickly lead to a downward spiral of poor mood, negative thinking, and ultimately poor physical and mental health.

Fortunately, the act of meditating can promote a relaxation response that switches off the excitatory neurotransmitters and reawaken the inhibitory ones, thus balancing your mood and calming your nervous system. In other words, you can attain the positive attitude and belief necessary for your brain to activate your natural pharmacy—all without the necessity for drugs or side effects.

That's not to say your mind can correct a serious medical condition without medical intervention, but it does suggest that meditation and mindfulness are a great complement to any treatment plan. Not only that, you can create positive lifestyle changes, whether it be weight loss, smoking cessation, pain management, stress reduction, learning acceleration and much more. Your life can be anything you dream it should be—the answer lies within the power of your own mind.

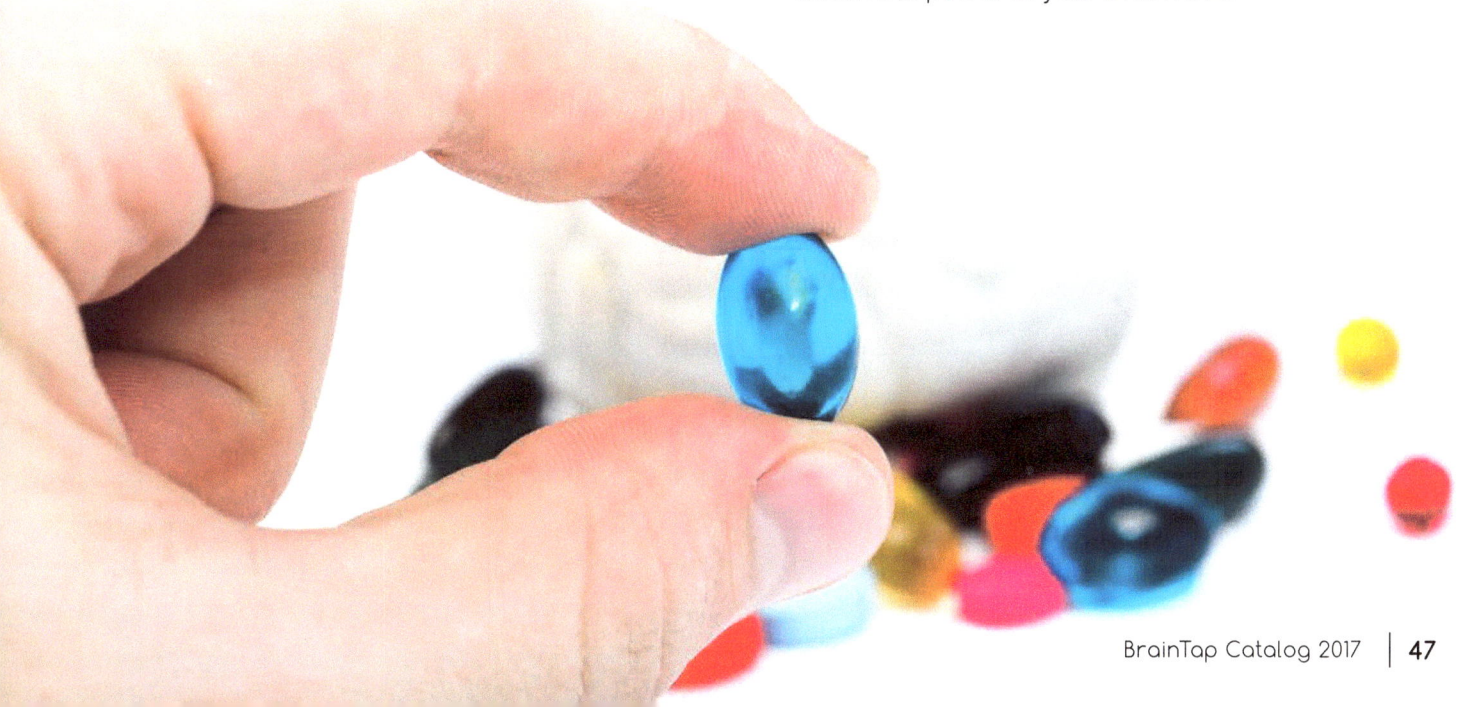

Pain

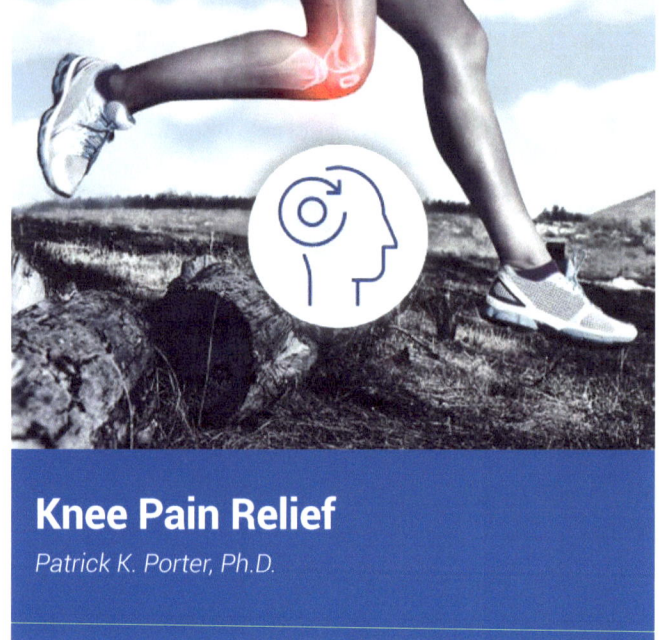

Knee Pain Relief
Patrick K. Porter, Ph.D.

Experiencing knee pain is not fun. During this series you will concentrate on eliminating any knee pain you have by changing your thoughts, avoiding foods that cause inflammation, and reducing your stress. You will find your symptoms beginning to alleviate while you relax and listen to this series designed specifically for knee pain relief.

KPAIN01 - SMT for Knee Pain Relief
Pain only exists in the brain, not the body. Learn how to refocus your thoughts to eliminate the pain that's holding you back.

KPAIN02 - Shedding the Light, Knee Pain Relief
Learn what is triggering your mind's reaction to the pain and how to refocus that energy to positive thinking.

KPAIN03 - Avoiding Foods that Trigger Knee Pain
Inflammation is caused by the food you eat. Create healthy eating habits that promote a stronger mind and body.

KPAIN04 - Reduce Stress and Reduce Knee Pain
Stress causes negative internal reactions and exacerbate pain. Reducing stress will calm your mind and body, therefore calming the pain your mind is experiencing.

KPAIN05 - Change is Key to Reducing Knee Pain
Lifestyle changes are necessary to decrease the actions that trigger knee pain. Learn how to make those changes without sacrificing your favorite activities.

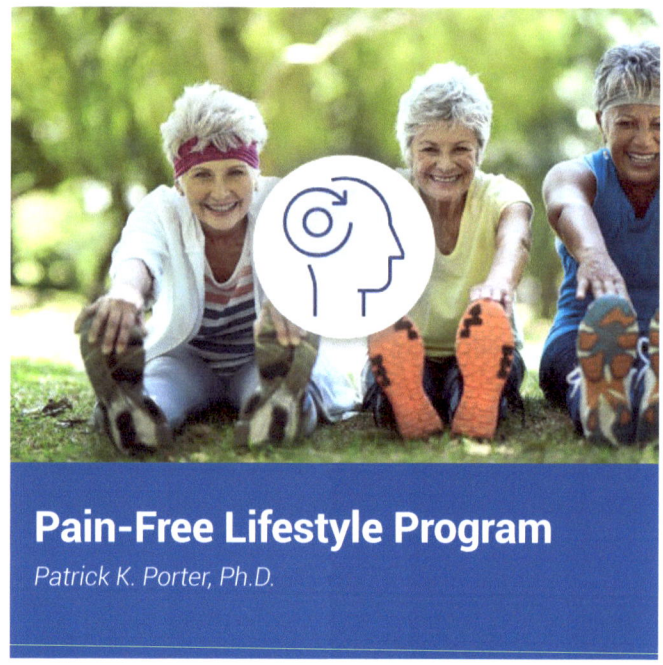

Pain-Free Lifestyle Program
Patrick K. Porter, Ph.D.

Persistent pain can have a costly impact on your life. It can lead to depression, loss of appetite, irritability, anger, loss of sleep, withdrawal from social interaction, and an inability to cope. Fortunately, with creative visualization and relaxation, pain can almost always be controlled. Visualization helps you eliminate pain while you relax, revitalize, and rejuvenate. You deserve to be free of your pain, and now you can be, thanks to visualization and the power of your own mind!

IMPORTANT! This series is intended to address habits and lifestyle choices while enhancing spiritual faith and should never be used in place of professional medical or mental health intervention. Never make medication changes without first consulting your doctor.

PF01 - Tapping into a Pain-Free Lifestyle
No one wants to deal with pain and discomfort. You will learn a simple exercise to transform pain into relaxation, and how to tap into your body's innate ability to heal itself.

PF02 - Activate Your Mental Pharmacy
Pain, fear, and anxiety all affect your mental being. In this session, you will unlock your body's natural pharmacy, releasing pain from your body and neutralizing all discomfort.

PF03 - Starting the Day Pain-Free
Transporting yourself to a pain-free state can seem difficult. In this motivational session, you'll learn to bury your pain in the past and awaken each morning pain-free.

PF04 - Developing A Pain-free Future
Train your brain to relax deeply with this session and help yourself break through the pain barrier. You will learn to go to sleep with certainty that you have the skills to awaken each and every day, free from discomfort.

PF05 - Removing Discomfort and Pain
Let the relaxing suggestions in this session, melt your pain away as you imagine yourself in a state of optimum health and harmony., learning that positive imaging can be your key to a lifetime of relief

PF06 - Train the Brain to Create Instant Anesthesia
Many of us wish we could naturally cure pain. Take these simple steps to link your body and mind, so that a free flow of natural pain relief will occur, even while you are awake, alert, and conscious.

PF07 - You Can Live Naturally Pain Free
This session provides a thorough summary of information on how to live naturally pain free, including breathing, visualization, and other relaxation techniques. You may even find that you can lessen or eliminate your need for pain medicine.

PF08 - Erase Chronic Pain and Enjoy Life Again
This session uses a compassionate visualization process that engages kindness towards yourself and your body. The emphasis is on letting acceptance happen, rather than trying to make it happen.

PF09 - Break the Emotional Bond to Physical Pain
Dr. Patrick Porter uses an advanced technique to help you flex your mind's pain-reducing muscles. You will focus on creating powerful, positive experiences that will create the remarkable brain chemicals that work with your body to eliminate discomfort.

PF10 - Develop a Healthy Pain-free Attitude
Pain is a signal to the body, and can be physical, emotional, mental, or all three. During this session, you will become aware of any resistance your body may have to becoming pain free, then release negativity and move you forward with a life-changing positive attitude.

PF11 - Mend Your Mind, Mend Your Body
You will use proven techniques for improving your self-esteem and assertiveness, helping you to feel better about yourself and plan your life more successfully. You will develop a the skills needed for a lifelong pain-free style of living.

PF12 - Develop Instant Pain Relief Triggers
You will learn useful tools for not only mastering the pain-free state, but for embracing a healthier lifestyle as well. This will help you relieve physical discomfort regardless of whether or not you are currently in pain.

PF13 - Generate the Relaxation Response to Remove Pain
As you relax, you will imagine a healing sanctuary that supports relaxation, and your mind's belief in your right to be healthy, strong, and vibrant.

Phobias

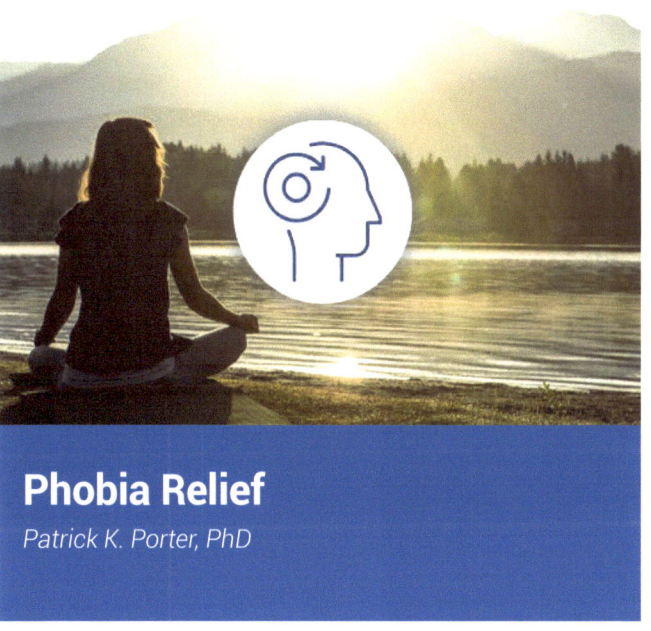

Phobia Relief
Patrick K. Porter, PhD

A phobia is a type of anxiety disorder that involves an irrational fear of a particular situation, an animal, a place, or a thing. Those with phobias will go to great lengths to avoid their fear, which is usually greater in their minds than in real life. The Fast Phobia Cure is probably the best known NLP technique. Dr. Patrick Porter will help you to use this technique to eliminate a minor fear or a full blown phobia.

PR01 - From Phobia to Personal Power
You will learn to let the power of your other-than-conscious help you to resolve the inner conflict and free your mind to return to a balanced state of acceptance.

PM

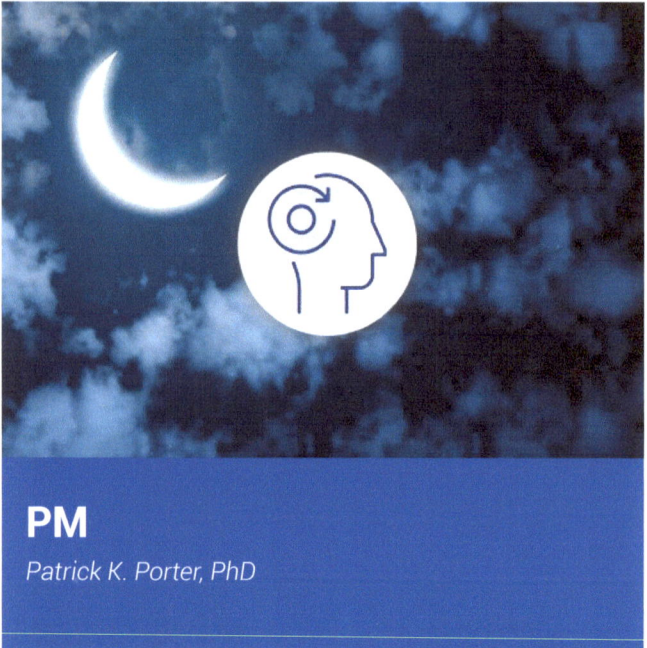

PM
Patrick K. Porter, PhD

PTSD

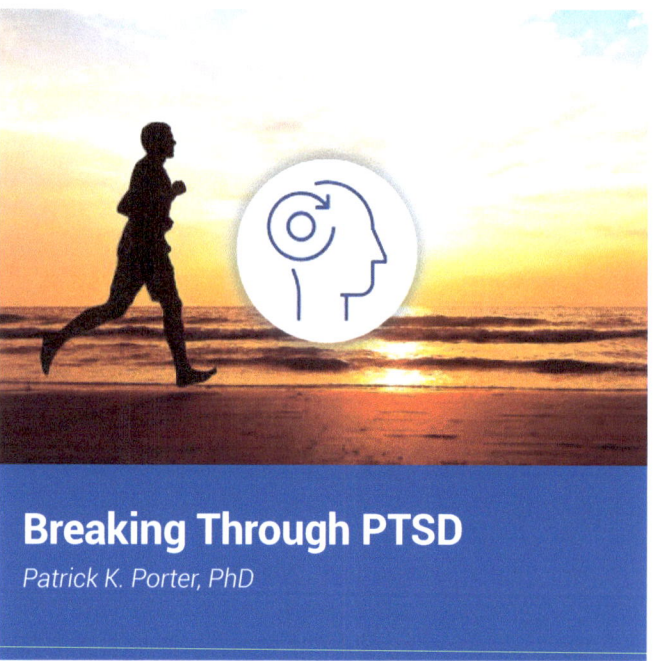

Breaking Through PTSD
Patrick K. Porter, PhD

PM01 - Focus In Dreamtime
Sleep often eludes us when our minds are cluttered with leftovers from the day's events. Dr. Porter created this session to help us enter into the deepest level of sleep by putting today's activities into perspective.

PM02 - Release Negativity
You will drift off into a deeply relaxing state of sleep where you focus on the positive, and eliminate the negative. The results will have you awakening with more energy and motivation to accomplish any task during the following day.

PM03 - Creating Your Success Timeline
You will drift off into a deeply rejuvenating sleep while the most powerful computer on earth continues to plan a timeline for success. You will be guided into restful sleep while your powerful mind plans success in your daily life.

> " *The truth is, we are all moving; some people are going forward, some backward, and others wherever advertisers tell them to go.*
> ~Patrick K Porter PhD

People who suffer from the effects of post-traumatic stress do so because they continue to re-experience the trauma in a way that affects them physically, mentally, and emotionally. PTSD sufferers tend to avoid places, people, or other things that remind them of the event and are unusually sensitive to normal life experiences. Although this condition has likely existed since human beings have endured trauma, in the past, advanced brainwave training was not available. But now you can learn to cope with the emotions resulting from a shocking, life-threatening, or otherwise highly unsafe experience and a new, more fulfilling lifestyle can be achieved. This breakthrough PTSD series is designed to help you release the past, create balance in the present, and build a compelling future.

IMPORTANT! This series is intended to address habits and lifestyle choices while enhancing spiritual faith and should never be used in place of professional medical or mental health intervention.

PTSD01 - Making Peace with Post Traumatic Stress Disorder
This introductory session will help you resolve the inner conflict from past experiences. Armed with this new way of thinking, you will create a new healing environment and begin to rebuild your life in powerful new ways.

PTSD02 – Reclaim Your Future after PTSD
When trauma happens, it can feel as if your future has been destroyed by a single past experience. In this session, you will learn to enter the powerful inner states of creativity and inventiveness, and start the rebuilding of social skills.

PTSD03 – Eliminate the Negative Effects of PTSD
Your mind is doing the best it can with the information it has at hand, but with this session you will take back your personal

power and write your own mental programs that bring back the joy, happiness, and wonder to your life.

PTSD04 – Putting the Pieces Together After Trauma
You will experience the galvanizing effect of looking at your situation from a fresh perspective. You will begin to mentally rebuild the inner relationships that bring trust, honesty, and self-confidence back into your life.

PTSD05 – Eliminate the Hidden Fear & Frustration After PTSD
With the seeds of hope, you can grow the strength of a giant redwood. You will discover what the great inventors of the past knew intuitively: if you have a problem in your life, your unconscious mind can solve it.

PTSD06 – Developing Hope as a Habit; Moving Beyond PTSD
Habits are programs that were written either by design or default. You will set up a series of positive triggers that will keep you focused on personal success and discover the power of living a life of choice not of chance.

PTSD07 – Using Forgiveness as a Resource
No one can change the events of the past. But you can change the way your mind recalls them. You will learn key phrases for changing your internal dialogue so that you can release the past and begin expecting good things to happen in your life again.

PTSD08 – Creating the Relaxation Response
You will learn the relaxation response as a way to feel the stress and then move through it to release the pressure. You will create a reservoir of relaxation that will inoculate you against everyday stress.

PTSD09 – Using the Theater of Your Mind to Reframe Your Past
Reframing involves looking at a situation in a new context. This session will allow you to separate the stimulus from the response so you are not subject to old patterns or beliefs and are free to create a new future.

> " *We get what we rehearse in life... not necessarily what we intend.*
> ~Patrick K Porter PhD

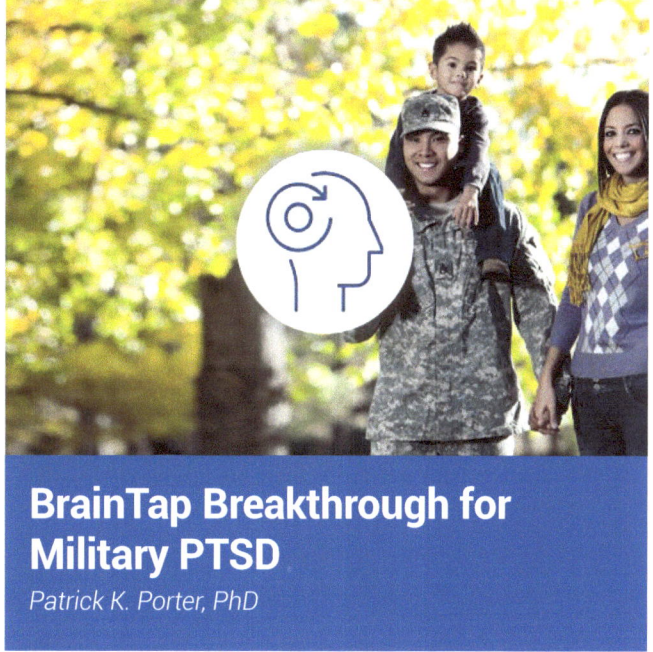

BrainTap Breakthrough for Military PTSD
Patrick K. Porter, PhD

People who suffer from the effects of post-traumatic stress do so because they continue to re-experience the trauma in a way that affects them physically, mentally, and emotionally. PTSD is very common among veterans, luckily this series is designed to assist with that. You will learn techniques to help you put your life back together after the traumatic experiences you encountered while in the military. You will learn to focus on the positive, and get back into the swing of civilian life by releasing the past, creating balance in the present, and building a compelling future.

IMPORTANT! This series is intended to address habits and lifestyle choices while enhancing spiritual faith and should never be used in place of professional medical or mental health intervention.

MPTSD01 - Making Peace with Life
This first session will help you resolve the inner conflict with the fight-or-flight response from the old triggers of past trauma. You will learn positive imagery that honors where you have been and helps you to get where you want to go.

MPTSD02 - Reclaim Your Emotions after PTSD
While past trauma could cause you to be quick to anger, you will learn effective ways to get moving and eliminate annoyances. You will let emotion (energy in motion) flow and feel your positive focus and concentration grow.

MPTSD03 - Turn Down the Volume on Negative
Mindful breathing is the key to turning down the effects of grief and guilt. You will take back your personal power, so you can reconnect emotionally, and bring back joy, happiness, and wonder to your life.

MPTSD04 - Reconnect with Life After Military Service
By connecting with others, you will release any remaining sorrow and begin to mentally rebuild the inner relationships that bring trust, honesty, and self-confidence back into your life.

MPTSD05 - Resolve the Conflict of Home Life and War
You might not feel like yourself without the rush of being in a combat zone and you may find it difficult to relax. This session will help bring the needed feeling of balance and purpose to your everyday life.

MPTSD06 - Develop Faith as a Habit
You will develope a feeling of being grounded through movement, touch, sight, smell, and taste. It comes down to everyday faith and creating a flow state, so the old disconnected feelings are replaced by purpose and personal power.

MPTSD07 - Use Forgiveness as a Resource
Even if you have seen comrades injured or killed, you can use the power of forgiveness to start the emotional healing. This session will help you release any survivor's guilt, and begin to expect good things to happen in your life again.

MPTSD08 - Safely Release Bottled Up Emotions
This session will help you assess your role in what happened and move on instead of reliving situations and punishing yourself. You will redirect your energy into honoring those you lost and finding positive ways to keep their memory alive.

MPTSD09 - Reframe Grief and Guilt and Be Free
With the stress of work and home, reframing the negative emotion of guilt will shift your energy to the positive. You will visualize positive outcomes, and have you back sleeping deeply and awakening in the days to come with a productive sense of wonder.

> " *Genius is attained with the realization that personal growth and the attainment of wisdom are the key ingredients to a successful life.*
>
> ~Patrick K Porter PhD

Public Speaking

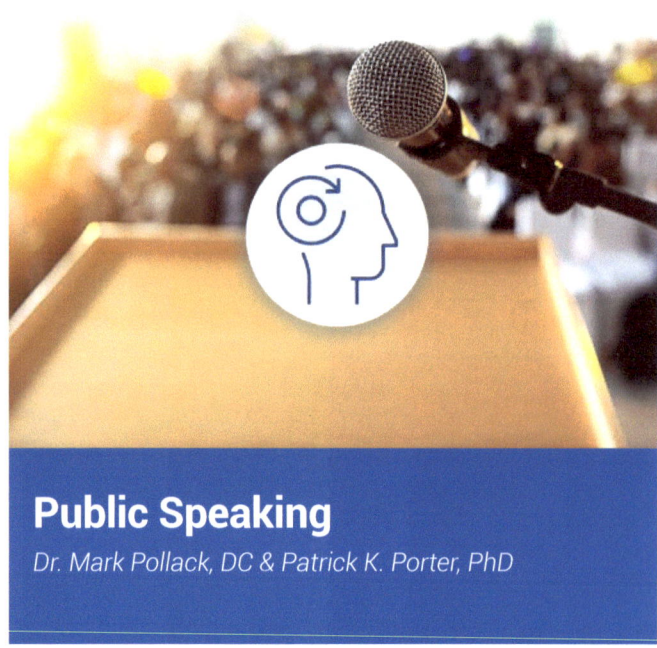

Public Speaking
Dr. Mark Pollack, DC & Patrick K. Porter, PhD

Public speaking comes natural for some, while for others is a frightening experience. If you find public speaking terrifying, you are not alone. This series will help ease that fear. You will learn techniques to help you feel more comfortable speaking in public. By the end of this series you will find yourself more relaxed than ever and fully equipped to speak to crowds of all sizes. This series is based on Dr. Mark Pollack's Wellness Speakers of America system.

WSA01 - Energy - Your Key to Opening the Doors of Business
Captivate your audience, keep them engaged, and learn how your energy on stage can move mountains.

WSA02 - Speaking is a Mind Game - Play it
It's not just about what you say, it's how you say it. This session teaches you how to utilize key words to get your desired outcomes.

WSA03 - Moving Beyond Phone Script Creation and Being 100% Present
Utilize the knowledge you've gained to use the phone as a tool, a stepping stone towards the end goal. Create comfort in phone conversations and capture the audience on the other end to further your relationship.

WSA04 - Master the Meeting, Master Your Event
Creative visualization is key to planning a professional, successful meeting or event. Learn how to focus on the end goal, leading to the execution of a flawless event.

WSA05 - Transforming Objections Into Opportunities
Not everything will go as planned, and that's ok. This session will teach you how to overcome objections and barriers, and how to make those objections work in your favor.

Sales Mastery

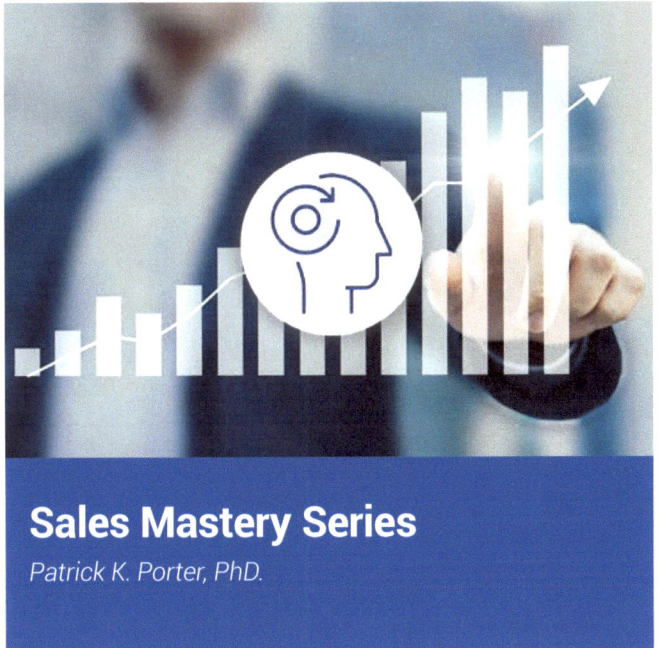

Sales Mastery Series
Patrick K. Porter, PhD.

Discover the powerful selling methods of sales masters. When you use this amazing series, you'll build your self-confidence, master your time, and learn to overcome all objections. By developing the skills and habits of successful sales masters, you'll realize your brighter sales future today.

SM01 - Sales Confidence through Self-Confidence
To have confidence in your sales skills, you need confidence in yourself. You will take control of your own self-confidence. You will organize your thoughts, put priorities in place, and take control of your sales.

SM02 - Supercharge Your Sales Skills
You already have all the abilities you need to become a sales superstar. This session will help you organize those resources to eliminate cold-call reluctance, and discover the secrets mastered by the true sales pros.

SM03 - Enjoying the Prospecting Game
This refreshing process teaches you to develop your infinite referral system, and make all the money you desire. When you approach sales with the mindset of a child, prospecting is not only easy, it's fun!

SM04 - Creating Your Sales Success Plan
Achieving success at sales can be difficult. You will discover quick, easy steps for implementing and working your personal success plan. When you have a plan, you create unlimited success in your sales career, as well as a balanced life at home.

SM05 - The Bigger the Goal, the Better the Result
Small thinking within your career and your life can affect your goals. You will use your creative mind to create bigger goals and better results. You will expand your ability to be flexible, even with difficult people.

SM06 - Build Your Personal Success Strategy
Creating balance in your life is not always easy. With this revitalizing session, you'll quickly wipe out procrastination and energize your daily sales activities. You will discover your dynamic self-image that's been waiting to shine.

SM07 - Rehearse Using Questions to Understand Your Prospect's Business
You will rehearse success scripts and see the unbelievable results play out. When you know the criteria your prospect uses to make decisions, it's easy to identify additional advantages to using your product or service.

SM08 - Fill the Need, Close the Sale
Closing the sale is the hardest part of the sales process for some. You will learn to quickly break the trust barrier and discover your prospect's needs so that closing the sale is as easy as taking a breath of fresh air.

SM09 - Eliminate Objections and Make the Sale
Your greatest sales obstacle lies in the mind of your prospect. This session trains your brain to listen for, and overcome objections before your prospects know they have them. Selling is easy when you use the simple laws of persuasion.

SM10 - Remove Your Competition from the Mind of Your Prospect
Competition plays a big role in making a sale. With this session you can get your prospect to eliminate your competition without you using a single negative word against them. It's easier than you think when you use these four simple steps.

SM11 - Going with the Flow: Closing Strategies & Objection Prevention
Objections are part of the sales game, but you'll learn how the power of "no" can actually help you reach your sales goals. In this session you will learn a simple three-step process to help you close the sale. You will be ready and able to close the most difficult prospect.

SM12 - Using Sales Reframes for Fun & Profit
Objections can be discouraging. In this session you will learn how to transition, or reframe a negative statement into a positive one with this motivating session. Even the most difficult sale is easy when you turn resistance into cooperation.

SM13- Tai Chi for the Sales Mind
Negative thoughts work against you and harmfully affect your sales performance. After this session you will be able to elevate your thoughts to the highest level. When your mind is on your side, anything is possible!

Sleep

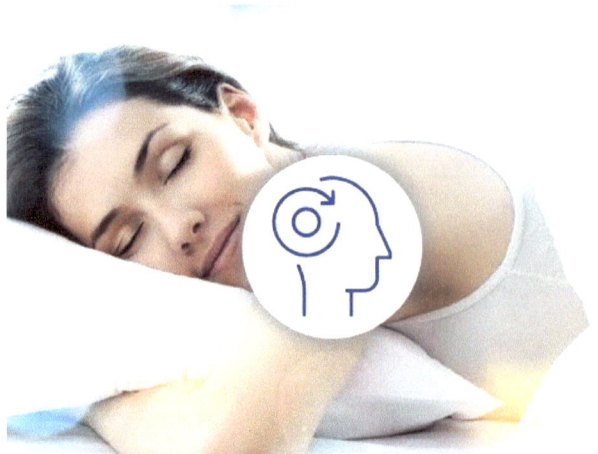

Healthy Sleep Habits Series
Patrick K. Porter, PhD.

When you don't get the optimal, restorative sleep your body needs, you may experience drowsiness, irritability, lack of concentration, and poor memory. The immune system may suffer as well. But there is a solution. In this series, Dr. Patrick Porter (PhD) will help you discover how to improve your sleep habits, restore natural sleep cycles, and provide you the energy and vitality you deserve each day.

IS01 – Sleep Deep and Awaken Recharged
Dr. Porter will guide you through the thought processes that will deliver the deepest states of relaxation and promote healthy, high-quality sleep.

IS02 – Planning a Restful Night's Sleep
You will learn to look forward to sleep by training your mind to think differently and remove any nervous tension at the approach of sundown, throughout the evening hours, and at bedtime.

IS03 – Making Peace with Your Body for Deep Restful Sleep
People who have poor sleep habits tend to try to control situations, people, and events that are beyond their control. You will release the unconscious need to react with fear, both consciously and unconsciously, about any situation that is not within your control.

IS04 - Sleep Deep & Let Go of Unwanted Fears Forever
You will learn the common physical changes that occur, such as floating, being in a trance, or a slowed heartbeat. You will learn to allow these changes to guide you into the deepest, most rejuvenating kind of sleep there is.

IS05 - Going with the Flow Day & Night
You will learn to think differently during the day so you can rid yourself of anxious thoughts and worries. You will no longer be mentally escalating negative thoughts and emotions during the day, allowing you to sleep comfortably all night long.

Smoking

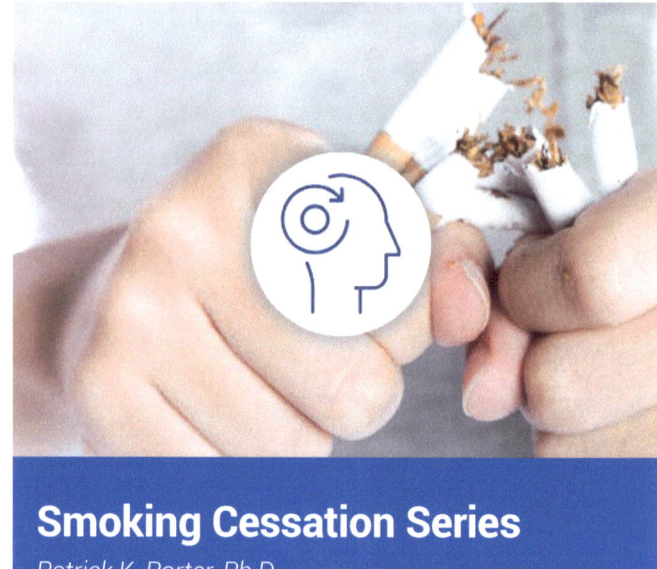

Smoking Cessation Series
Patrick K. Porter, Ph.D.

Kicking your smoking habit doesn't get any easier or more fun than this! When you use Dr. Patrick Porter's proven strategies, you'll find that making this life-saving change comes about naturally. These sessions will help you extinguish the stress and frustration associated with quitting smoking, and you'll conquer your cravings like the tens of thousands of others who have used his techniques. You will learn to stay calm so you can easily and comfortably vanquish the old urge for cigarettes. Breaking the chains that have bound you to cigarettes has never been easier—now that you have made the choice to live your life tobacco-free and to start living the life of your dreams!

SS01 - Making the Decision to Be A Non-Smoker
You will learn about the cleansing power of your own mind, and use it to take a mental shower that will wipe away all thoughts of tobacco and gladly make the decision to be tobacco-free for life!

SS02 - Making Peace with Your Mind
The smoker of the past will make peace with the clean air breather of the future and create a new, vibrant you!

SS03 - Plan Your Life as a Non-Smoker
This motivating session will allow you to remember to forget cigarettes forever. You'll awaken convinced being a nonsmoker is as easy as taking a breath of fresh air!

SS04 - Freedom from Tobacco At Work
This process is specifically designed to help you learn new ways to handle daily breaks, drive time, and times when your co-workers might be smoking around you.

SS05 - Craving-Free/Tobacco-Free
Cravings will become a thing of the past as you employ the world's greatest computer... your human mind!

SS06 - Rid Your Mind of Stress & Frustration
Dr. Patrick Porter has trained thousands to use these success strategies to eliminate stress and frustration, and now he is going to help you.

SS07 - Feel the Flow and Let Go - Tobacco-Free
You will learn techniques of self-discipline and self-confidence that will train you to remain 100% tobacco-free for the rest of your life.

SS08 - Count Down to Being Tobacco-Free
This session will have you creating new triggers for health. As you develop self-discipline and self-confidence, a new life filled with health and abundance becomes yours.

SS09 - Total Relaxation for The Non-Smoker
You will use the power of relaxation to transform stress into positive energy that will help you accomplish your goals. It's easy when you use your mind to simply relax away your cravings.

SS10 - Thinking Like a Non-Smoker
As you allow your mind to return to its natural way of thinking, it will be as natural as your heart beat to remain tobacco-free.

SS11 – So Hum Tobacco-Free
You will discover the power of selective thinking so you can remove your cravings and accentuate the positive of living tobacco-free.

SS12 - Problem Solving as A Non-Smoker
Stress is one of the main reasons people smoke. In this session, you learn to creatively handle stress and create solutions that will make it easy to stay tobacco-free.

SS13 - Healthy Mind for A Tobacco-Free Lifestyle
Learn this quick three-step process for thinking and acting healthfully and you'll find that de-stressing and conquering deadly habits like smoking is easy.

The Secret to a Perfect Night's Sleep!

Those who suffer from sleeplessness know its debilitating effects. Lack of sleep causes weight gain, depression and anxiety. It can throw off hormonal balance and hinder the immune system.

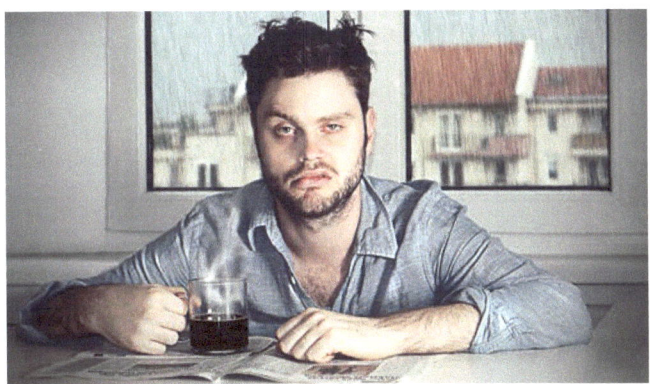

Sleep deprivation can have the same hazardous effects as being legally drunk. Getting less than 6 hours a night can affect coordination, reaction time and judgment, posing "a very serious risk."
~Occupational and Environmental Medicine

We've all experienced sleep issues due to the stress in our daily lives. Whether it's work, relationship issues, financial problems or just life in general, statistics show that more than 30% of the US population suffers from sleep deprivation. It's gotten so bad that the CDC recently pronounced, "Insufficient sleep is a public health epidemic."

According to a study in the *International Journal of Psychophysiology*, evolution may be to blame. Chinese researchers discovered that our bodies are primed to stay awake when we perceive threats, and nighttime stress may amplify this response. In other words, our brain perceived the dark of night as a more threatening time because that's when our ancestors faced the most threats. When we feel stress, our brains think we're in danger and keeps us on high alert, diminishing the possibility of a good night's sleep.

Your body was not designed to remain in high states of stress all the time. Sadly, most people spend the better part of their day experiencing super-stress. Your brain copes by generating high intensity brain waves that overpower the brain waves designed to calm you, especially at night. Once your brain becomes used to this hyper alert state, it can become very difficult to wind down.

Fortunately, the BrainTap headset is a great way to sleep more deeply and awaken refreshed. Its gentle light and tone pulses bring down the rapid brain waves that cause sleeplessness while activating the brain waves that make you feel calm, balanced and happy. It also helps get rid of the negative mind chatter that often causes restlessness and helps you develop positive new thought patterns to manage stress, get focused, feel more confident, and enjoy an overall sense of wellbeing.

For more information or a complimentary trial of the BrainTap headset, please ask your health provider or visit **www.braintaptechnology.com** to search for an authorized BrainTap provider near you.

Sports

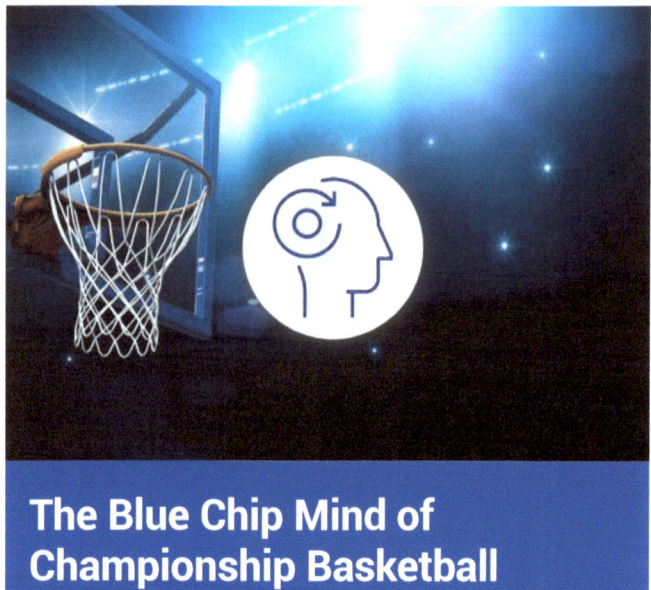

The Blue Chip Mind of Championship Basketball
With Anthony Simms & Patrick K. Porter, Ph.D.

After former Olympian and NBA player Anthony Simms experienced Dr. Patrick Porter's techniques, he recognized it as a way for the youths he mentors to build the intrinsic motivation and commitment of a champion. He saw visualization as a solution for the many young competitors who could never afford a personal sports psychologist, and as a way for athletes to easily practice mental rehearsal, a proven method for improving skills and instilling muscle memory.

BCB00 - Demo: Communication of Champions
This is a visualization for staying in the moment, using a technique for alerting your teammates of your opponent's noticeable patterns. After this session, you will be able to unleash your excellence on the court.

BCB01 - Developing the High Values of a Champion
As an Olympic athlete and professional player, Anthony found that the values you have in life are the values you bring to the court. You will learn to keep your highest values present so you stay focused and motivated.

BCB02 - Reading your Opponent For Championship Play
Anthony says that in a split second you need to know whether the player is tall or short, left- or right-handed, fast or slow, a power or finesse player, tough or soft. You will learn this skill through a a breakthrough technique called modeling.

BCB03 - Developing the Pre-Game Mind of a Champion
You will gain the ability to read your opponent's strengths and weaknesses and then go into battle mode. These mental drills that will have you thinking positively and focusing on success before you ever step on the court.

BCB04 - Developing the Post-Game Mind of a Champion
This session will give you the skills needed to review your performance with no regrets or judgments. The post-game mind puts you into a state of preparedness for your next game and your daily routine.

BCB05 - Using the Science of Observation to Create Your Winning Skills
You will master your understanding of rotation, arch, precision entry through the rim, and motion of release. Now when you watch great shooters, you will be in the habit of building your basketball IQ.

BCB06 - Moving from Setting Goals and Dreaming to Being a Champion
When Anthony is asked what one final word a champion truly understands, that word is commitment. You will ignite a burning desire, and an all-out laser focus on your championship goals.

BCB07 - Moving from a Novice to a Champion with Lightning Speed
Champions know they must transform weaknesses into strengths. Time spent listening to this session is time spent mastering the skills of a champion from the inside out.

BCB08 - Understanding the Metaphysics of Basketball
You will find that inner place where you move faster, jump higher, and meet the rim with ease. As you progress through this session, you will see yourself delivering offensive and defensive actions effortlessly.

BCB09 - Blue Chip Basketball
This session will help you identify with the blue chip athletes who aspire to perform at their optimum level on and off the court each and every day.

BCB10 - Standing on the Shoulders of Champions
You will apply the science of observation by mentally hanging out with champions in order to learn to duplicate their winning advantage. You will find yourself humble while at the same time burning with the desire to be a champion.

BCB11 - Commanding the Emotional Game of Basketball
Aggression, intensity, and self-control are words used to describe champions. This session will have you in command of yourself and your opponent at all times.

BCB12 - Developing Your Coachable Mind
You will learn to keep an open mind and let new information empower you. Your new, coachable mind will be hungry for the information that will raise your level of skill and achievement.

BCB13 - Activating Laser Focus
Learn to have laser-like focus so you stay in the zone and everything works. You will practice focus in a new way and will develop your own activities that trigger the focus response.

BrainTap Your Way to the Top of Your Sport

Michael Phelps is the most decorated Olympian of all time with a total of **28 medals.** Phelps holds the all-time records for Olympic gold medals (23), Olympic gold medals in individual events (13), and Olympic medals in individual events (16).

Bob Bowman, who's been Phelps' coach since he was a teen, taught Phelps **visualization** as a part of his mental training. Bowman had Phelps watch a "mental videotape" of his races every day before he went to sleep and when he woke up in the morning. Phelps would visualize every aspect of swimming a successful race, starting from his release at the blocks and culminating in a winning celebration.

But visualization isn't just for elite athletes like Phelps, it can be used regularly as a part of your ongoing training program with significant results.

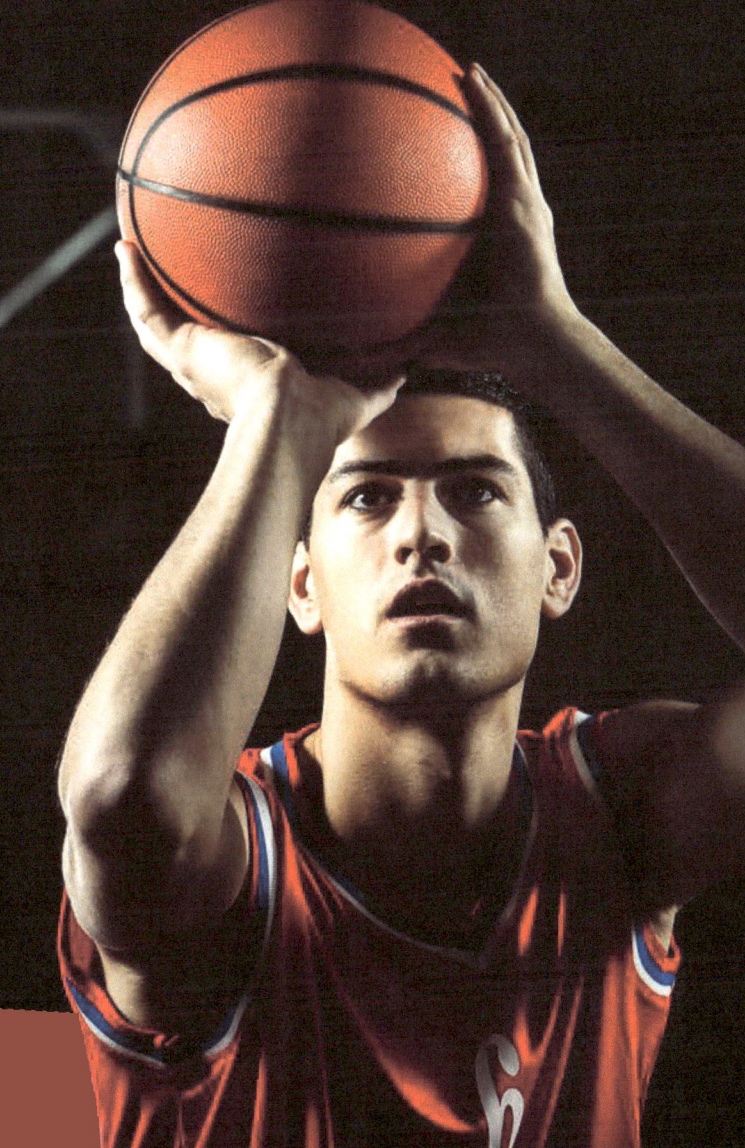

This benefit was discovered by physiologist Edmund Jacobson when he had subjects visualize physical activities. Using sensitive detection instruments, he discovered subtle but very real movements in the muscles that correspond to the movement the muscles would make if they were actually performing the imagined activity.

Further research revealed that a person who consistently visualizes a certain physical skill develops **muscle memory,** which helps when they physically engage in the activity. A related study by Australian psychologist Alan Richardson confirmed the reality of the phenomenon.

Richardson chose three groups of students at random. None had ever practiced visualization. The first group practiced free throws every day for 20 days. The second and third group shot free throws on the first and twentieth day. Members of the third group spent 20 minutes every day visualizing free throws. When the students in group 3 missed a free throw, they mentally practiced making it before moving on to the next free throw.

On the twentieth day Richardson measured the percentage of improvement in each group. The group that practiced daily improved 24 percent. The second group showed no improvement. The third group, which had physically practiced no more than the second, did 23 percent better—almost as well as the first group.

In Richardson's paper on the experiment, published in Research Quarterly, it was pointed out that the most effective visualization occurs when the individual who is visualizing feels, hears and sees what they are doing. For example, **feeling** the ball leaving their hands, **hearing** the ball bouncing and **seeing** the shot go through the net.

When competitive athletes slip into their zone, everything seems to work just right. Dr. Patrick Porter will help you get to that place where everything comes together. With the **SportZone Series,** you will learn to visualize yourself into a flow state, your own personal zone, so you can stay on top of your game. The zone is as easy to access as a deep breath once you have mastered the mental keys.

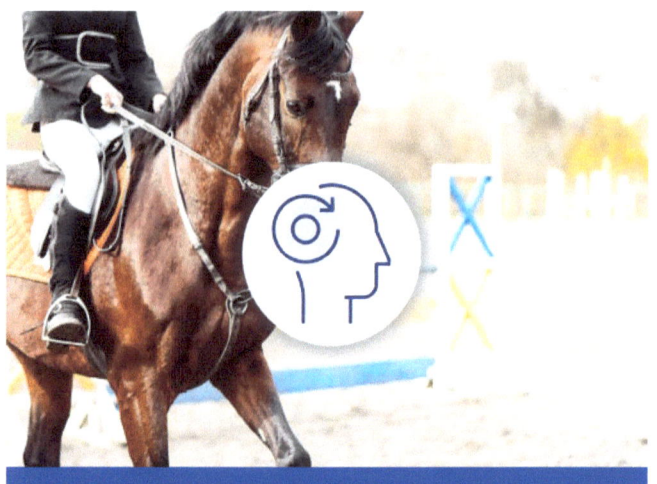

Equestrian
Dr. Wendy Coren

There is an equestrian zone that riders slip into when they are aligned with their equine partner and the course flows naturally before them. Join Dr. Wendy Coren as she guides you to that place within, your personal zone, where you will build the attitude, confidence, and skills of an equestrian master.

EME01 - Riding In The Zone
You will be guided to your personal zone, where everything is naturally right and blue is the outcome. All it takes is a deep breath to enter your zone once you have mastered the mental cues.

EME02 - Moving Forward
What would happen if your restraints to greatness were removed? No blinders. No draw reins. No doubt. You can simply move forward to accomplishing your boldest dreams by changing perspective and developing positive aids for success.

EME03 - Building The Attitude For Altitude
The ability to jump higher and farther than ever before is accessible. You have the ability and agility to succeed. You will build the attitude to propel you onwards and upwards.

EME04 - Riding Best Under Pressure
Creating the skills to respond to pressure with performance is what this exercise is all about. Transform pressure to perfection.

EME05 - Think Like A Grand Prix Equestrian
Grand prix riders train the mind, body and spirit. In this session, you will learn to think and process the way champions do. Soon the grand prix mindset will be second nature to you.

EME06 - Dual Voice Ride Your Pace
You know exactly what pace to ride for whatever event you choose. Now you can make it real first in your mind, then in the ring. You will program that cadence for the perfect pace into your performance every time.

EME07 - As You Ride So Shall You Be
The lessons you learn to create the ideal ride are the lessons that apply to your life. Applying those skills effortlessly is the outcome of this session—cool, confident, collected and successful.

EME08 - Feeding The Equestrian Brain Step By Step
Becoming the equestrian you choose to be is a process. As you follow the sequence for success, you will train your inner world to manifest in your outer world.

EME09 - Balancing Your Life
Success and happiness come together when each part of your unique personality gets its fair share of intention and attention. This session will bring balance to your life.

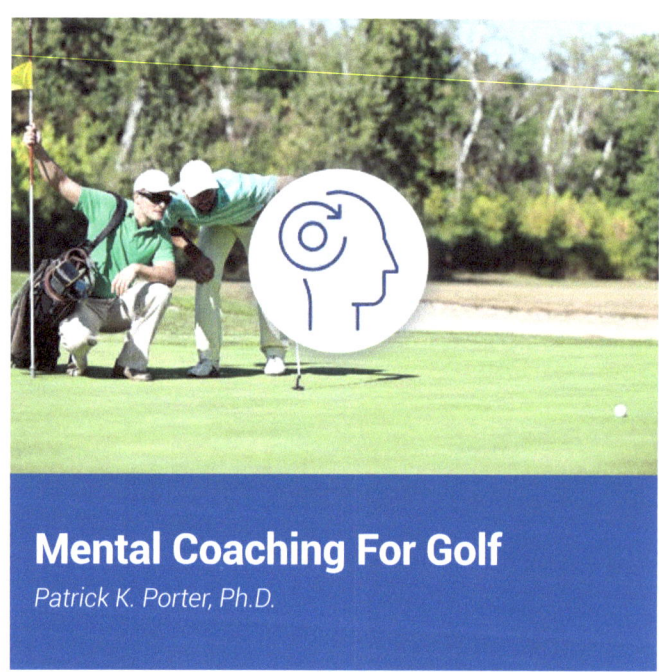

Mental Coaching For Golf
Patrick K. Porter, Ph.D.

Efficient golfers know how to relax and let their minds take over. Now, thanks to these creative visualization sessions, you'll learn to see yourself as a calm, confident golfer. You deserve to take pleasure in your time on the course. You'll finally be able to let go of frustration and focus on every stroke—meaning you'll not only play better, but you'll also enjoy the game more than ever!

GF01 - Optimize the Risk Zone for Golf
You will practice each swing, letting go of negative thoughts, and allowing the clubs to do what they were designed to do—send the ball straight to the target.

GF02 - Develop the Attitude of a Champion
You'll no longer waste time feeling distracted, over-analyzing your

game, or blaming the conditions of the course. Instead, you'll admire the trajectory of a well-struck drive, a clean chip shot, or a perfectly sunk putt, as you play and think like a champion!

GF03 - Concentration: Your Key To Consistency
You'll learn to block out distractions, focus like never before, and discover the concentration that will help you play the best golf of your life!

GF04 - Discover the Confidence of a Tiger
Learn to face any part of the course with complete self-assurance. You have good instincts—you just have to trust them. From now on, you will use the positive power of your mind.

GF05 - Tame Your Tempo and Score
Sit back, relax, and let this refreshing session instill the skills you need to look at your game from the outside in. You will be able to set your perfect tempo, lower your score and, most importantly, enjoy your game to the fullest.

GF06 - Rehearse Excellence and Eliminate Execution Errors
You will learn to visualize the ideal shot every time you address the ball. You will rehearse the feeling of accomplishment you get from making all the right choices at the tee, then be able to stand back and enjoy your perfectly executed drive.

GF07 - Release Pressure and Tension
You will learn to release pressure and tension under any circumstances. Loosen up, take a deep breath, and let the pressure roll away as you experience your ultimate relaxation both on and off the course.

GF08 Gain Finesse and Lower Your Score
You will learn techniques that will prove to you how five minutes of visualization can be equal to two hours of physical practice. With this mental edge you will have more fun on the course than ever before!

GF09 Golf is a Mind Game... Play It!
You will imagine what it's like to take a ride inside the mind of the golfers you most admire. You will be guided into the realm of infinite possibility where you can master each and every phase of the game you love.

GF10 Master the Course, Master Your Round
You will learn to master the game by knowing your strengths and weaknesses. Now you can immediately improve your handicap by playing smarter and staying in control, even in the most challenging situations.

GF11 Erase Nervousness and Perform Under Pressure
Dr. Patrick Porter will show you how a positive mental attitude will help to reduce nervousness and naturally reduce your score. Relaxation tips will help you release any anger or frustration before you address the ball.

GF12 Three Easy Steps to Great Golf in Any Situation
Putting together a great game is all about routine. This session takes you from a good stance to a polished mental attitude and beyond. You'll use these keys to lower your score, and enjoy it more as you open your mind to the possibilities.

GF13 Golfing in Dream Time... Your Key to the Ultimate Swing
It's been said that what the mind can conceive and believe, the body will achieve. In this session you will mentally rehearse your goals so the unseen forces of the mind will bring them into reality!

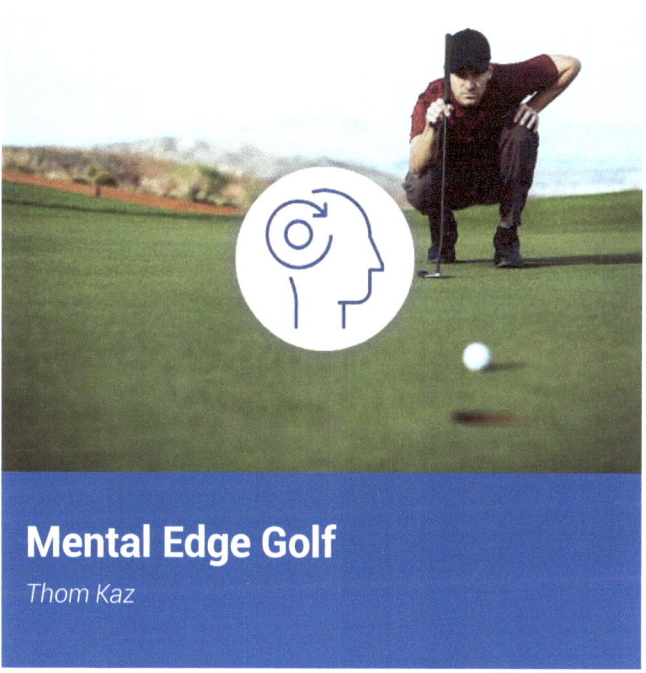

Mental Edge Golf
Thom Kaz

This program is designed to help program your instincts to play more effectively, and enter the state of mind and body called the zone. Entering into the zone makes it easier to play the game. You will be focused on peak performance and learn to relax in order to achieve this level of performance. You will learn the difference between process focus and outcome focus, and how to perfect your skills in order to putt like a pro.

TKG01 - Develop the Perfect Swing
Some people say their practice swing is just fine, but when it comes to real play it's not the same. With this session you will learn to direct your focus at will in order to develop your perfect swing.

TKG02 - Focus and Concentration
To be a high performer at any skill in life, you need to know how to focus at the right time to focus on the task at hand. During this session you will learn how to ignore any outside distractions and focus on the flow.

TKG03 - Hitting Over Hazards
When hitting over a hazard it is important to hit your normal shot. With this session you will learn that whether you're hitting over a steep incline or over a body of water you need to remain focused on your shot.

TKG04 - Putt Like a Pro
Negative thinking can ruin your game. During this session you will learn to become one with your putt in order to improve your game.

TKG05 - Teeing off with Confidence
When you are in the game, past failures and successes do not matter. You should be focused on right now in order to tee with confidence.

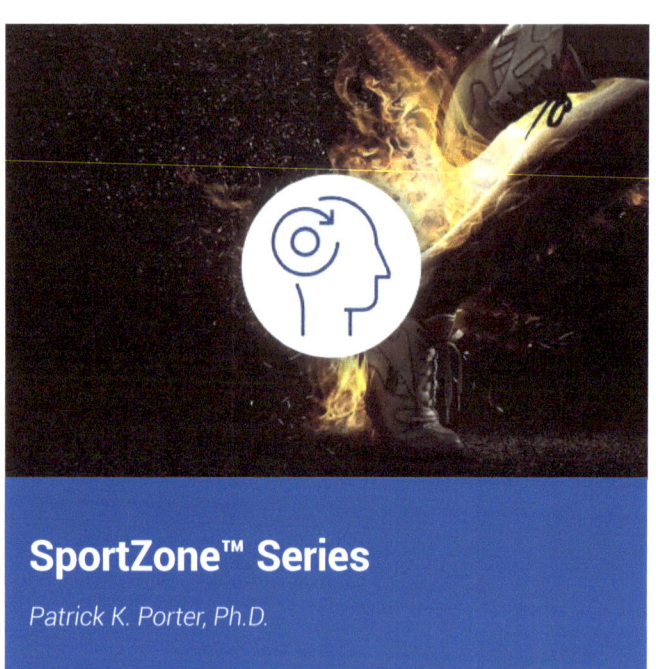

SportZone™ Series
Patrick K. Porter, Ph.D.

Visualization for sports performance is nothing new to top competitors—athletes from Tiger Woods to diver Greg Louganis, and a variety of Olympians have used visualization to bring about optimal performance, overcome self-doubt, and give themselves a seemingly unfair advantage over their competition. Now the SportZone series can work for any athlete, from junior competitors to weekend enthusiasts. Yes, you can get more out of your sport and, in the process, get more out of life.

SZ01 – Using the "Zone" in Your Sport
When competitive athletes slip into their "zone" everything seems to work just right. With this session you'll learn to put yourself into a state of "flow," your own personal "zone," so you can stay on top of your game.

SZ02 – Control Your Emotions and Master Your Sport
It has been said that he who angers you conquers you; this is true even if the person who angers you is you! You will learn a powerful technique for keeping your emotions under control, and no longer give your power away to others.

SZ03 – Super-Charge Your Self-Confidence
What would happen if you could cast out all doubt about your success? You will no longer hope, believe, or wish it to be so—you will know it to be so! You will be able to super-charge your self-confidence after listening to this session.

SZ04 – Psych Yourself Up! – and Perform Your Best Under Pressure
You will be given the specific step-by-step strategies you need to perform your best under pressure, eliminating "outcome anxiety," and ending with your willingness to visualize success.

SZ05 – The Secrets of Mental Mentoring Revealed!
Everyone has an inner champion. With this breakthrough session you will awaken yours and train it to go to work for you around the clock, even while you work, play, and sleep!

SZ06 – Set Goals Like the Pros
Self discipline can be hard to master. In this session, Dr. Patrick Porter teaches you the secrets of full-sensory goal setting. You will develop the concentration to focus on daily, weekly, and monthly goals.

SZ07 – Feel the Pressure and Win!
Dr. Patrick Porter will help you learn ways to transform negative pressure into an iron will. Your other-than-conscious will then use that newfound inner strength to create results for you in sports and in life.

SZ08 – Build Desire, Drive & Perseverance
You will create a compelling future and draw that future to you like a powerful magnet. You will build resources you need most, whether it's on the tee-box, a tennis court, a football field, or your own backyard.

SZ09 – Think Like a Champion
In this session, Dr. Patrick Porter will reveal all the leadership skills of a professional athlete so you, too, can have the confidence and determination you need when you need it the most.

SZ10 - Lessons in Sports, Lessons in Life
You will design your own creativity generator, build problem-solving skills, work through specific scenarios, and see yourself achieving every one of your life goals.

Stress

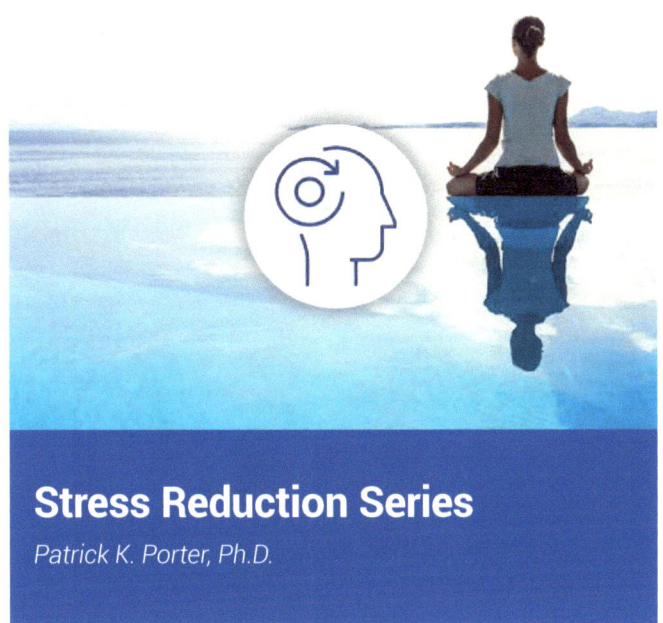

Stress Reduction Series
Patrick K. Porter, Ph.D.

Stress is the most pervasive malady of our time. The effects on our health, productivity, and quality of life are more devastating than most people care to admit. Luckily, you've just found the solution. Visualization can help you see yourself as the healthy, happy, optimistic person you'd prefer to be. With this new image, your fears and frustrations fade away, your anxiety vanishes, and you no longer let small things stress you.

SR01 - Create Your Enchanted Forest for Stress Reduction
Follow along as Dr. Patrick Porter guides you through your personal enchanted forest—a quiet, serene place where you have nothing to do but relax. You'll return from your magical forest filled with positive feelings, able to enjoy and express your true inner peace.

SR02 - Create Your Mountaintop Retreat for Stress Reduction
Say goodbye to all stress and confusion as you take a trip to this breathtaking mountaintop retreat. By using your mind, relaxing your body will become as comfortable and automatic as breathing. The stress of everyday life will melt away so you awaken renewed.

SR03 - Experience Dream-time and Achieve Your Goals
You will walk along your dream beach, as well as change past failures into triumphs—even meet your future self to see the successes you've achieved.

SR04 - Putting Future Events Into Perspective
Dr. Patrick Porter will show you the benefits of having a healthy picture of the future. You'll put your future into perspective and learn creative ways to live your life without unhealthy stress.

SR05 - Reducing Uncertainty And Doubt
You will be guided to discover hidden talents that will help you reduce or eliminate doubt. You will train your brain to yield spontaneous relaxation, helping you to create a healthy body.

SR06 - Eliminating Negative Thinking
You will experience the healing force of your mind. Once your own healing power is working within your body, you will build a shield of protection against anything that is less than vibrant health for you.

SR07 - Making Peace With Your Past
You will learn to forgive, forget, and move on with a healthy body and attitude. With the power of forgiveness on your side, the unseen forces of your mind will create radiant health.

SR08 - Rehearse Mental Harmony for Physical Health
With this powerful process you will actively use mental housecleaning techniques to cleanse your mind, and help you to unleash your body's natural ability to create perfect health.

SR09 - Stress-free Mind, Healthy Body
You will learn how your thoughts, actions, and beliefs shape your body. Sit back, relax, and enjoy discovering these amazing secrets for cultivating a healthy mind, and enjoy life in a healthy, strong body.

SR10 - Developing Spontaneous Relaxation
Sometimes you need to relax and get focused right now! You will train your other-than-conscious mind to soak up a series of soothing creative visualization and relaxation processes that will yield relaxed and positive thoughts on demand.

SR11 - Free Your Mind & Experience Your Healthy Body
We think thousands of thoughts every day. Learn how to cast out the negative, listen to the positive, and unleash your mind's healing force. You will build a shield of protection against anything that might stop you from experiencing radiant good health.

SR12 - Creating a Life of Vibrant Health
You will learn how easy it is to release any hurts from your past that might hold you back from your commitment to health. This process engages the healing graces that allow you to forgive, forget, and move on with a healthy body and attitude.

SR13 - Allowing a Life of Health & Abundance
You will be guided through the garden in your mind where you will train your other-than-conscious to focus on action, success, and health. You will learn new and creative ways to live your life without the need for stress.

Wealth

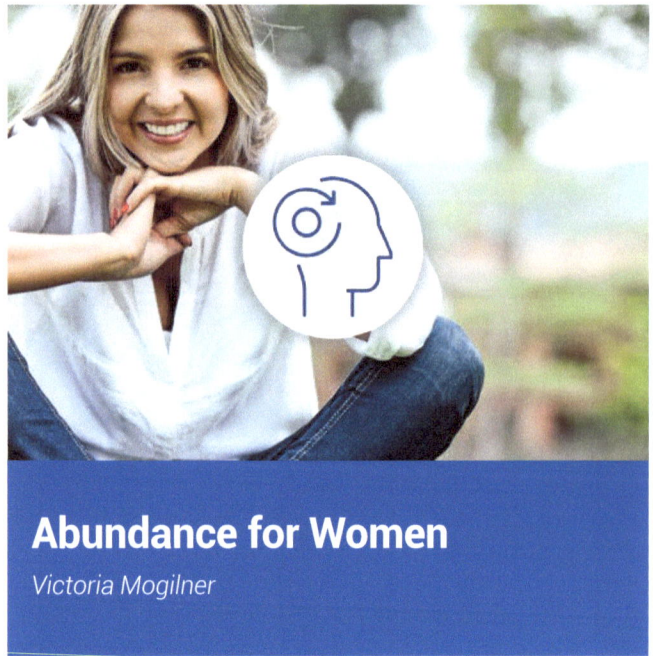

Abundance for Women
Victoria Mogilner

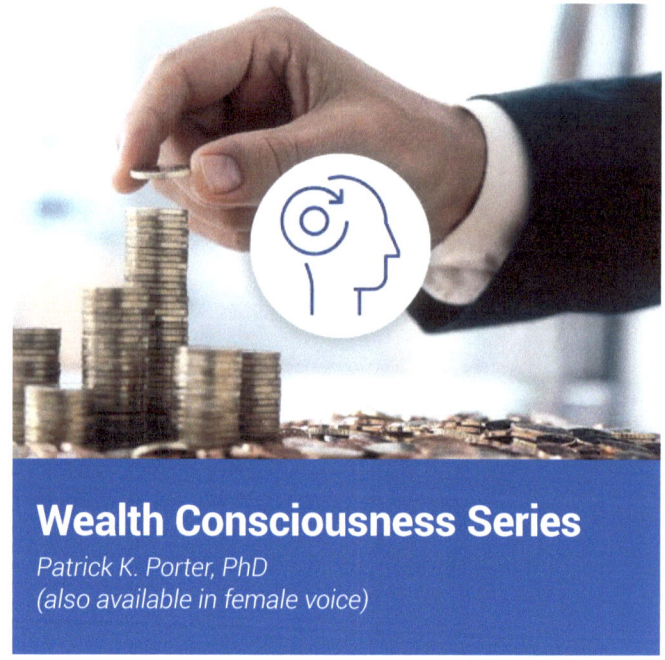

Wealth Consciousness Series
Patrick K. Porter, PhD
(also available in female voice)

VM01 - Abundance for Women
Victoria Mogliner takes you on a journey of creative visualization that teaches you how to gain success and balance in all aspects of your life, allowing you to flourish.

VM02 - Loving Yourself from the Inside Out
Learn that success starts on the inside. Let Victoria Mogliner teach you how to strengthen your love for yourself internally, so that you can take on the world externally.

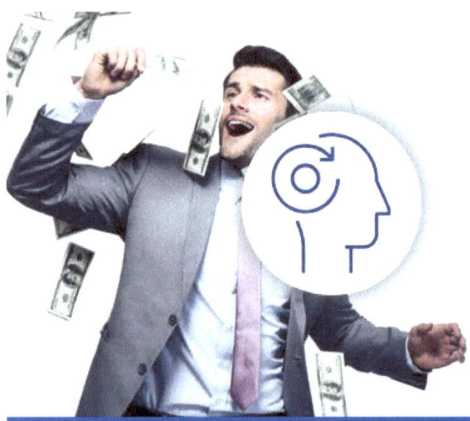

Busting Loose From the Money Game
Robert Scheinfeld and Patrick K Porter, PhD.

BLFM01 - Busting Loose From the Money Game - The Process
From best-selling author, coach, and entrepreneur, Robert Scheinfeld, learn the invisible blockages keeping you from reaching your success and ultimate freedom. Break free and enjoy the feeling of true fulfillment.

Inspired by the principles of Napoleon Hill's Think and Grow Rich.

"Imagination is the workshop of your mind, capable of turning mind energy into accomplishment and wealth."
— Napoleon Hill

WC01 - Start Each Day with Purpose and Passion
This session will guide you in using the power of intention to focus on the success and prosperity you desire. You will begin reaching the level of success you have always imagined.

WC02 - Commit to a Life Spent with Like-Minded People
In this session you will activate what Napoleon Hill termed the "third mind," or group intelligence. With each visit to this level of the mind, your mastermind alignment will grow stronger.

WC03 - Trusting the Power of Infinite Intelligence
Poverty is a fear that controls many people. You will visualize the thoughts and actions that show you how to become successful. You will begin noticing wealth and riches flowing into your life.

WC04 - Exceed Expectations - Serve Others, Serve Yourself
You will become motivated by a help others mindset. This feeling of service will magnetize wealth and abundance to you.

WC05 - Transmit a Pleasing Personality to the World
You will tap into your true radiant personality. It's easy to draw wealth and abundance to you when you show up with a pleasing personality.

WC06 - Harness the Power of Personal Initiative
You will gain the behaviors of a motivated self-starter. You will notice personal initiatives will inspire you to greater success.

WC07 - Claim Your Right to a Positive Mental Attitude
You will uncover the positive attitude that resides within. You will eliminate unproductive thoughts, enhance your relationships, and balance your life.

WC08 - Radiate Enthusiasm - Your Key to Success Consciousness
This session will allow you to tap into your desire to win and the physical energy that we call enthusiasm. You will be fueled by desire, which creates enthusiasm, which fuels determination, and leads to success.

WC09 - Grasp the Power of Thought and Ordain Your Destiny
You will enhance your self-discipline, which Napoleon Hill called, "taking possession of one's mind." This new habit will allow you to take charge of your life as your positive new thoughts create a new world around you.

WC10 - Tuning Into Infinite Intelligence for Accurate Thinking
Infinite intelligence can be a tough concept to grasp. During this session you will learn to trust your connection with infinite intelligence. You will be able to examine information, build discernment, and make the decisions that shape your destiny.

WC11 - Awaken the Seeds of Achievement
Awaken the sleeping seeds of greatness that will carry you to heights you might never dreamed possible. You will learn to fix your attention on what you want, instead of what you don't want.

WC12 - Harnessing the Power of Cooperative Effort
You will move beyond mastermind groups into a coordinated effort to work with a team spirit. You will learn about your definiteness of purpose and absolute harmony.

WC13 - Find the Solution to Any Problem
This session will allow you to see problems for what they really are and dwell on solutions instead of problems. You will realize problems are temporary setbacks and stepping stones to success.

WC14 - Tap Into The Creative Vision of Infinite Intelligence
While listening to this session you will make the inner connection with the guiding force that lets you accomplish the impossible. You will notice how wealth flows to those who work smarter, not harder.

WC15 - Health Consciousness, Wealth Consciousness
There is a universal truth that what the mind dreams about the body brings about. In this process, you will plan a life of wealth, health, and abundance from the inside out.

WC16 - Employ the Power of Time for Wealth Consciousness
In this session you will discover how to use assertiveness and diplomacy to get what you want. You will keep the dream stealers and time bandits out of your life so you can keep your eye on the prize and enjoy the ride to riches.

WC17 - Build Your Wealth One Habit at a Time
This session will show you how making positive choices becomes a driving power in your life as you master the power of thought. Your other-then-conscious mind will become your guide in building unlimited wealth.

Weight Loss

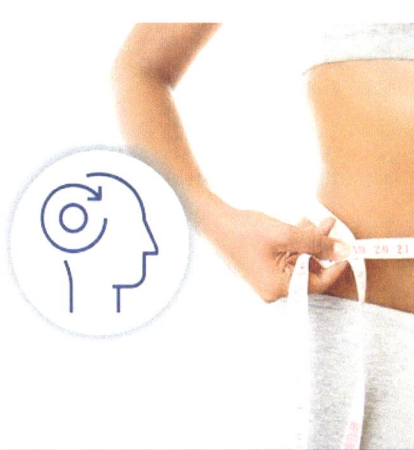

Blissful Body Meditation Course
Jennie Carlson

This meditation series is designed to help you realize you have the power within yourself to heal your body. During these brief sessions you will reminisce on your past in order to provide a better future for yourself. All you need to do is sit back and relax, while allowing Jennie Carlson to guide you through this blissful body meditation course.

BBM01 - Introduction Blissful Body Meditation Course (No Lights)
This introductory session explains how to listen to this series. This series will help you delve into your past and heal any disconnects within your body, mind, and spirit. You will be able to connect with your present, and your future.

BBM02 - Plug In Connect Protect
In a world of so much external noise and distractions it's easy to feel scattered and overwhelmed. With this session you will plug into your support system, connect to higher consciousness, and protect yourself from negative energy.

BBM03 - Healing Past Hurt
No one had a perfect childhood. We all had defining moments that have shaped how we function in the present. In this session you will learn to heal these past hurts and change the negative patterns that are holding you back from reaching your potential.

BBM04 - Future Grid
Sometimes our goals seem so big and scary we're not sure we can accomplish them. You will discover your future guide and hear their words of wisdom and encouragement for moving forward in a big way.

BBM05 - Past, Present, Future
In this session, you will learn to take the lessons you've learned from the past, and the wisdom from your future guide, to propel you to greatness in the present moment.

BBM06 - Healing Body
Sometimes, the idea we have of our body isn't true and doesn't serve us, in fact it causes disease to stay longer than necessary. You will learn to see your body as perfect and whole for complete healing to take place.

BBM07 - Releasing Worries
We live in a stress filled world with deadlines and mountains of responsibility. Take a break from these stresses and allow yourself to relax with this session. You will learn to rid yourself of any worries you may have.

BBM08 - I Love You, I Forgive You, Thank You
Self criticism can weigh you down. In this session you will learn to step back from the self-criticism and invoke compassion instead. This is an ultimate practice in gratitude for the body and all it does for you.

BBM09 - Congrats (No Lights)
You have completed the meditation course. Hopefully you have learned some useful techniques to help you heal. You now know that you have the answers within yourself to heal.

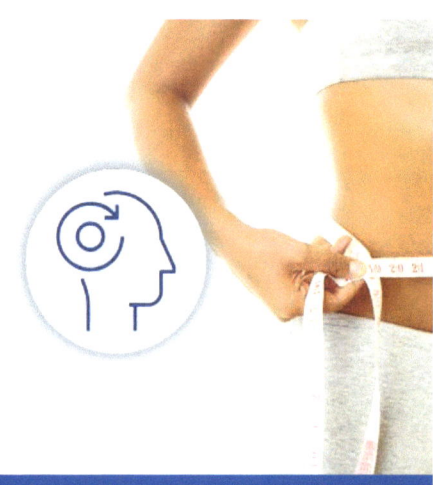

Habits of Naturally Thin People
Patrick K. Porter, Ph.D.

Now you can design the body you want and the life you love. Once you have a new image of yourself, everything else changes—junk food and fast food lose their appeal, healthy foods become desirable, and you eat only when you're hungry. With this system you will overcome common weight loss mistakes, learn to eat, and think like a naturally thin person, conquer cravings, and increase your self-confidence. Each week you will take another step toward a lifetime of healthy living; losing weight is the natural byproduct of these changes. While the average diet lasts just 72 hours and focuses on depriving you of the foods you love, Dr. Patrick Porter supercharges your weight loss motivation with these powerful visualization sessions. You will eliminate the problem where it started—your own mind. There is simply no easier way to lose weight than visualization.

WL01 - Safely Speeding Up Weight Loss
You'll learn to safely speed up weight loss by thinking, acting, and responding like a naturally thin person. Your sense of worth will improve when you discover and use inner resources you never even knew you had.

WL02 - Simple Steps for Self-Confidence for Weight Control
Discover your bright and compelling future—a future where all your physical, mental, and emotional goals have been reached. Gain new confidence in your healthy behaviors, aware that your future is filled with infinite possibilities!

WL03 - Eliminate the Gain/Loss Cycle
You will let go of the past, because the past no longer controls you. The present is your most powerful moment, and in the present you're free to make the choices that will help you realize and maintain your natural and ideal weight forever.

WL04 - Producing Success One Thought at a Time
Eliminate the negative thoughts, patterns, and beliefs that have been keeping you from reaching your goals. As you release negative thoughts, and excess weight, you'll free yourself to enjoy more joy and success than you ever thought possible!

WL05 - Sunrise Agreement
As you experience this session by Dr. Patrick Porter, your old habits and new desires will communicate and create a contract for success. With this "Sunrise Agreement," you'll awaken knowing every day is a new day, given to you to create the changes you desire.

WL06 - Create Your Weight Loss Support Team
You will use the power of your mind to help you to build a caring and supportive team that will improve every relationship. With this type of attitude you will create all the support you need to reach your goals.

WL07 - Developing Positive Eating Patterns
You'll mentally journey back to a time when you enjoyed doing the best for your body. You'll find yourself more comfortable and confident each day, effortlessly eating the right foods at the right times.

WL08 - Turn Up Your Fat-Burning Thermostat
You will rehearse the proven steps that allow your body to convert into a fat burning machine naturally. These simple tips will help increase your metabolic rate and show you how to keep your weight off.

WL09 - Motivation for Monday Morning
Monday mornings seem to be the ideal time to start changing your life. With this inspiring session you'll learn to recapture that beginning-of-the-week motivation, and use it every day of the week.

WL10 - Using Your Mind's Eye for Weight-Loss Success
Enter the theater of your mind and watch your own weight-loss success take place before your eyes. Success follows you when you solve the problems of your past with solutions you see in your present and future.

WL11 - Stop Dieting and Start Living
Your mind has a natural ability for removing mental obstacles to your weight loss. You will discover why appetite is of the mind and hunger is of the body. Returning to your natural weight is easy when you plan a lifetime of healthy thoughts and actions.

WL12 - Exercising is Energizing
Wouldn't you love to have fun exercising? With this session you'll develop the thoughts and skills of a person who naturally loves to exercise. You'll see excellence in the naturally-thin people around you and develop the same abilities in your own life.

WL13 - Take Back Control of Your Appetite
The average person gains up to four pounds a year. This session is developed to break this cycle. You will discover why true happiness starts when you eat to live, and eliminate any thought of living to eat.

WL14 - Break the Chains that Keep You from Ultimate Health
You will find it easy to create a new reality where you are no longer imprisoned by negative thoughts, patterns or beliefs. You will open the treasure chest of your natural talents, and awaken yourself to the freedom of today.

WL15 - Stay Fit Through Healthy Eating Patterns
You will eliminate the habits that caused you to gain weight, and then choose the habits and behaviors you need to remain naturally thin. It's easy to stay on track when you forget about dieting and make lifestyle changes instead.

WL16 - Extinguish Junk Food Cravings
You will visualize simple steps that transform your appetite so you'll crave the healthy foods that keep you thin. You will take back control and leave your unhealthy eating patterns in the past.

WL17 - Quick Tips To Lose Weight Even If You Eat Out Everyday
Eating out can be a treat and a timesaver. Someone else does the cooking and there are no dishes to do. In this session you will discover how to take back control of your health by taking control of your food choices.

WL18 - Eliminate The Traps Associated With Dieting
Dieting traps can vary from Monday morning blues to Friday night fever—traps almost every dieter has fallen prey to. Discover how easy it is to avoid these dieting traps by using your mind to rehearse your best intentions.

WL19 - Visualize & Realize a Lifetime of Weight Loss Success
No one wants to have to diet over and over again. You will reframe the old patterns that held you back in the past so you can lose your weight once and for all.

WL20 - Making the Connection for Permanent Weight Loss
You will discover the secrets of naturally thin people and how to implement them in your life for permanent weight loss. With this connection, true health will be yours and negative thoughts about yourself will never again control you.

WL21 - Eliminate the Desire for Sugar & Chocolate
You will focus on creating the desire for positive, life-giving foods that are fresh and alive. From this new mindset, you'll respond to foods with health in mind. You will realize that nothing tastes as good as thin feels!

WL22 - Self Control And Radiant Health
When you learn to erase all doubt from your mind, it's easy to stay purposeful and on track with your health goals. You will learn to display discipline and confidence while having fun.

WL23 - Asking For What You Need and Getting What You Want
If you've had trouble communicating your desires in the past, it will become easy for you using these exciting new communication skills. You will visualize yourself communicating with others with assertiveness and confidence.

WL24 - Choosing Habits That Keep You Naturally-Thin
You will unleash the power of selective thinking and learn to choose the foods and activities that are healthiest for your body. You will build a lifestyle that will support you in staying naturally thin.

WL25 - Exercise - Your Key To Lasting Health & Vitality
Imagine how good you will feel as you burn fat, build muscle, and sculpt the body you want. With this session you will ignite your enthusiasm for health and exercise. You will mentally rehearse your active new lifestyle where exercise is fun and enjoyable.

WL26 - Breezing Through the Weekends Naturally Thin
Now you can end the weekly weight loss roller coaster. This session is specially designed to keep your goals in high gear even on the weekend. Imagine the joy of starting the week with unlimited confidence!

WL27 - Free Yourself from Overweight Thinking
As you develop your naturally thin mindset, it's important to unlock the gates of your mind and release the past. You will build your new body image and envision the future where you are healthy, confident, slim and attractive.

WL28 - Make Exercise An Automatic Part Of Your Life
Studies show that people who learn to enjoy exercise are far more likely to maintain their weight loss. You will find powerful ways to boost your metabolism, which is your key to lasting energy. When exercise is automatic and fun you create a more active lifestyle.

WL29 - Sugar Busters ... How to Have Your Sweets and Lose Weight Too
Even naturally thin people eat sweets from time to time. Now you can too, without guilt or shame and without derailing your weight loss progress.

WL30 - Learn the 10 to 1 Method for Giving Your Body What It Needs
You will learn to use instant triggers to help you throughout the day to think and eat like a naturally thin person so you can give your body exactly what it needs effortlessly.

WL31 - Make Your Daily Activities Your Daily Motivation
Your daily routine can become dull and boring after a while. You will visualize how your daily routines can turn into excitement as you mentally cleanse your mind and body.

WL32 - Make Your Motivation to Exercise Sizzle!
Exercise is fun when you feel motivated. You'll be guided to develop an effective and lasting exercise program. You'll turn fat into lean body mass by using your mind to make exercise fun.

WL33 - Building Your Self-confidence and Self-esteem
If you've ever failed at dieting, you've lived the disappointment that follows. Now you will erase all that negativity and discover fun and creative ways to transform your thoughts, actions and beliefs into those of a healthy, happy you.

WL34 - Unlocking Your Innate Intelligence to Recreate Your Body
When you make peace with your body, you won't have to force it to do anything. You will learn the difference between power and force. You'll then find it easy to ride the power wave of change, making it easy to think and eat the way thin people do.

WL35 - Using Assertiveness in Weight Control
It's easy to say yes or no when you are steadfastly focused on your health goals. Experience progressive relaxation while you plan your life and be set you free from the emotional roller coaster of the lose/gain cycle.

WL36 - Finding the Exercise You Like and the Time to Do It
Design a healthy environment where exercise fits into a busy lifestyle. You will learn to create balance in your home and work life so you'll be thinking and acting like a thin person in no time.

WL37 - Accept and Love Your Body
Give your body the loving care it needs and deserves. When you learn to build a positive relationship with yourself by loving and accepting your body, making good choices becomes easy.

WL38 - Gain Power Over Your Appetite
You will learn to recognize the difference between appetite and hunger so you can make food choices from a place of self-empowerment.

WL39 - Staying on Track with Your Transition to Thinness
Everyday you are bombarded with over 50,000 messages, each one prompting you to think or act in certain ways! Dr. Porter will help you stay focused on your transition to a healthier, happier lifestyle.

WL40 - Eliminate Your Weight Loss Enemies For Good
Learn to eliminate the old enemies that kept you trapped in negative programming of the past. Whether it's food, family, friends, or your own self-talk, you will relax and allow your mind to work out success on your terms.

WL41 - Plan a Healthy Home and Workplace
Creating balance in your home, work, and personal life can be overbearing. You will eliminate any destructive or limited behaviors that may otherwise sabotage your weight loss goals and learn to motivate yourself.

WL42 Supercharge Your Self-image
You will learn powerful techniques that empower you to enjoy fresh and alive foods as much, or more than the old junk foods of the past. You will learn to savor the flavors in fresh, natural foods.

WL43 Eliminate Fear And Stay Naturally Thin
The primary factor in disappointing weight-loss results is fear-of-failure. Dr. Porter will help you to eliminate this fear-of-failure thinking so that keeping your weight off becomes effortless.

WL44 Mental Toughness for Weight Management
You will create a rock-solid attitude about being naturally thin and staying at your natural and ideal weight. Learn to generate resources when and where you need them to accomplish your health goals.

WL45 Increasing Self-Esteem and Optimism
Self-esteem is an inside job. You will create the habit of optimism, which will help you conquer fear, frustration, and anxiety, while experiencing a peaceful mental vacation.

WL46 Conquering Cravings for Sugar and Unhealthy Fats
Whether your cravings are related to stress, hormones, habit, or your own self-talk, relax and allow your other-than-conscious mind to work out success on your terms.

WL47 Removing the Unwanted Appetite of the Past
You will learn to recognize true hunger, which is a different feeling from appetite. You will learn how to unlock the power of possibility thinking, and feel the habits of a naturally thin person grow within you.

WL48 Healthy Eating During the Holidays
Why suffer or feel deprived when everyone else is having a good time? When you focus your mind on the positive experiences, and easily eat and think like a naturally thin person, your holidays will be a delightful experience once again.

WL49 Put Your New Year's Resolutions on Overdrive
Many of us never follow through with New Year's Resolutions. You will tap into the limitless motivation within you to stay on track, build unstoppable resolve, and accomplish your resolutions with ease.

WL50 Giving Thanks and Staying Slim
The average person gains weight over the holidays. You can use this session to create healthy holidays, and overcome the poor eating habits and associated stress. You will be able to eat less and enjoy the holidays more.

WL51 Celebrating Parties and Picnics Guilt-Free
Why stress at parties while everyone else is having fun? Relax with this session and you'll soon find yourself enjoying good times with friends and family without the worry, deprivation, or guilt of the past.

WL52 Keeping It Off with a Naturally Thin Mindset
Imagine your life after you find fun ways of focusing on yourself at your natural and healthy weight. By developing an

awareness of who you truly are, it will be easy for you to eat and think as a naturally thin person.

WL53 Eliminating the Fear in Losing Weight
The thought of losing weight can seem like an uphill battle. In this session you will learn to eliminate the fear holding you back from achieving your weight loss goals.

WL54 Changing Your Thinking
You will learn to make losing weight naturally your number one priority. You will positively change your thinking in order to reach your ideal weight.

WL55 Tips and Tricks for Making and Keeping New Year's Resolutions
Trying to stick with your New Year's Resolutions can be difficult. During this session, you will learn to use positivity to make, and keep your New Year's Resolutions.

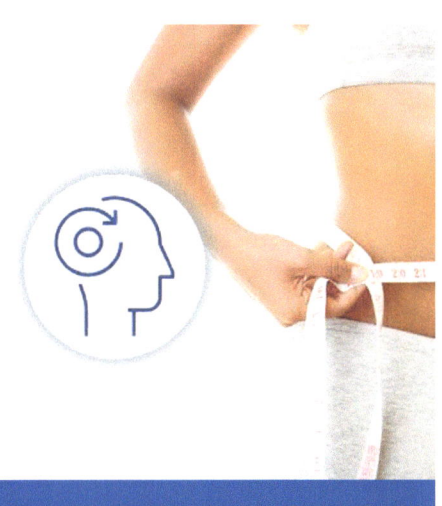

HS Weight Loss
Patrick K. Porter, PhD

HealthSource is known as America's chiropractor, and this series is based on their whole-health philosophy. They understand how hard maintaining your health can be, because when you're working long hours, and juggling just about everything else in between, it's easy to let your health take a back seat to your life. We were tired of seeing patient after patient being held back by their weight, with no cure in sight. This series is designed to help you continuously focus on your goals, and keep the weight off.

HSWC01 - Breaking the Chains of Weight Loss Resistance Syndrome
Trying to portion out your food can be difficult. In this session you will be able to look at food and think as a naturally thin person, and eat only the amount you need.

HSWC02 - Creating A Diet That Works for You
Diets can be hard to stick with. With this session you will learn to create, and stick with a diet that fits your specific needs.

HSWC03 - Supercharge Your Joy for Exercise
Everyone doesn't find exercise enjoyable. Dr. Patrick Porter will help you tap into your joy for exercising, so you will become interested in your weight loss process.

HSWC04 - Turn Your Body Into A Fat Burning Machine
With this session you will focus on eating a balanced meal and drinking plenty of water in order to transform your body into a fat burning machine.

HSWC05 - Living Your Life As A Naturally Thin Person
Negative thoughts can affect how you view yourself. You will learn how to eat right while maintaining a positive attitude.

HSWC06 - Eliminate Overweight Behaviors
In this session you will learn that the past is the past, and the future is open to all possibilities. However, you will focus on right now, and remain optimistic in order to realize your full potential.

HSWC07 - Erase Triggers that Caused the Weight in the First Place
With this session Dr. Porter will help you escape old triggers of the past. you will open your mind to the possibility that there are greater possibilities.

HSWC08 - Developing the HealthSource Mindset for Life
You will learn to find ways to remain comfortable even in stressful situations around difficult people. You will focus on immediate solutions when problems arise in regards to your health.

HSWC09 - Planning Your Life Naturally Thin
Imagine yourself a year from today at your target weight. This is what you will visualize in this session, and you will realize you have the tools and resources you need to succeed.

HSWC10 - The Plan Works so Work the Plan
You will realize with this session that the plan works when you only eat when you're hungry, and eat just that amount. You will learn to make health one of your top priorities.

HSWC11 - Making the Lasting Connection
During this session you will learn how to love, appreciate, and honor yourself. You will also learn to stay on track towards the direction of your goals.

HSWC12 - Unlock Your Creative Genius
With this session you will learn to build a plan to focus on your strengths, improve your weaknesses, and succeed effortlessly.

HSWC13 - Harnessing the Power of Commitment
During this session you will rethink your commitment to health, and experience the lasting weight loss you desire.

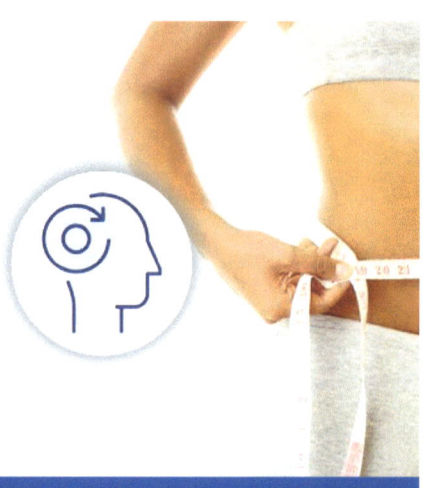

Lipo-Light Ultimate Body Contouring Program
Patrick K. Porter, PhD

Each title in the series is specifically designed to enrich your Lipo-Light experience while motivating you to succeed. You will experience a significant reduction in stress, better sleep, and a positive mental attitude. You'll develop the motivation and drive to exercise, eat right, and get the most out of your Lipo-Light Treatments. There is no better mind/body combination for weight reduction than the Lipo-Light with BrainTap!

LLU01 - Visualize your Healthy Body Makeover
You'll learn to master your mind so you can keep your toned and well-shaped body for a lifetime.

LLU02 - Detoxify & Stimulate Your Fat-burning Hormones
You will learn the benefits of detoxifying the body to help you trigger fat burning between sessions for optimum results.

LLU03 - Stimulate Fat Release
You will be deeply relaxing and training your brain to trigger the fat burning hormones that are released during periods of deep relaxation.

LLU04 - Exercise to Super-charge Fat Burning
Build your motivation and drive to continue your exercise program for immediate and visible slimming and toning in the areas you want.

LLU05 - Eliminate Trouble Spots Diet and Exercise Can't Reach
You will visualize unwanted fat being released from trouble spots and be empowered to follow through with your toning and shaping program for lasting results.

LLU06 - Water: Your Key to Maximum Results
The fastest way to develop optimum brain activity is by drinking water, which leads to excellent decision-making. You will discover the benefits of daily detoxifying, and the healing effects of water.

LLU07 - Healthy Eating Skills
You will learn creative ways to eat, think, and respond to life as a naturally thin person. You will be able to build these skills into your lifestyle naturally.

LLU08 - Super-charge Fat Burning While You Sleep
You will regulate your internal clock so you sleep better and awaken revitalized. You will learn techniques that have helped millions of people sleep deeply without trying.

LLU09 - Eliminate Stress-Food Triggers
Trigger foods are a part of life, so learning to say no without stress is key for lasting weight loss results. You will visualize meeting your trigger environment and emotions in positive ways.

LLU10 - Maintain Your Ultimate Body Shape
You will retrain your brain to monitor your daily activity and eliminate the problem where it all started—in your mind. You will be able to look forward to lasting results.

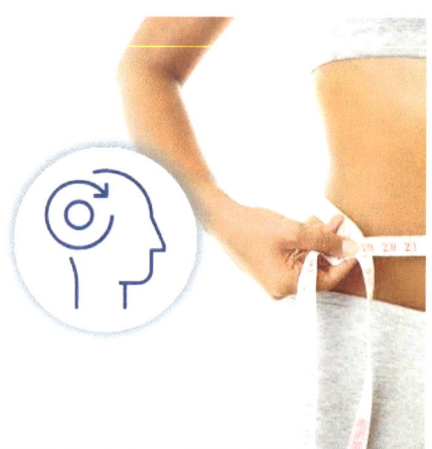

Weight Loss through Consciousness
Cheree Ann Porter

Cheree Porter took inspiration from her father, Patrick K. Porter, Ph.D. and developed a visualization series based on the thought that it is important to gain an understanding of oneself and one's place in the world in order to succeed at losing weight. The series includes sessions teaching the importance of exercise and eating right while awakening an inner sense of self with a firm, positive view of the world we live in.

WJGF01 - Embrace Your Powerful Self Esteem
You may not enjoy eating healthy. In this session you will be motivated to eat healthier by eating more fruits and vegetables per day, and drinking plenty of water. By doing this, you will get rid of any unwanted and unnecessary weight.

WJGF02 - Conjuring Faster Weight Loss Wiccan Journey
Many people wish to lose weight fast. You will visualize your body at its natural weight, and let go of any negative emotion, and focus on positivity. You will learn to eat healthy foods to stimulate natural fat burning in your body.

WJGF03 - Banish Junk Food Cravings
Eating too much junk food can cause you to act in ways unlike yourself. With this session, you will change the way you think of junk food. You will focus on fresh foods, and they will become more important to you.

WJGF04 - Evoke the Power to Exercise
Exercising is dreadful for some. During this session, you will let go of any limited beliefs that have prevented you from exercising. It will become enjoyable to you, allowing you to lose weight faster.

WJGF05 - Evoking Weight Loss and Health Success
With this session, you will eliminate any confusion associated with weight loss, and allow your body to make healthy choices. You will learn to eat the amount necessary to get healthy and remain healthy.

WJGF06 - Living in Infinite Health
Many people don't like dieting. With this session you will change your attitude about dieting, by focusing on a healthy lifestyle. You will be eating to provide yourself with health, vitality, and harmony.

WJGF07 - Conjure Your Healthy Life
Creating a healthy life begins with a thought, which will turn into a behavior. You will learn how this behavior will show up at the right place and the right time for you, allowing you to conjure a healthy lifestyle.

Writing

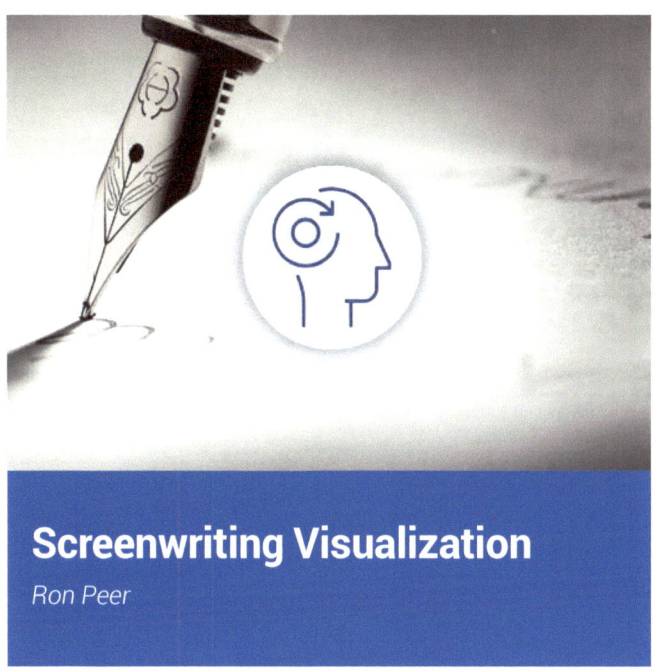

Screenwriting Visualization
Ron Peer

RP01 - Screenwriting Visualization
Screenwriting can be a daunting task. Ron Peer will help you get over your fear of believing your ideas are not good enough, and tap into the great screenwriter you were destined to be.

> *If you consider the true value of time, you'll find out you're already prosperous.*
> ~Patrick K Porter PhD

What the media has to say about Self-Mastery Technology...

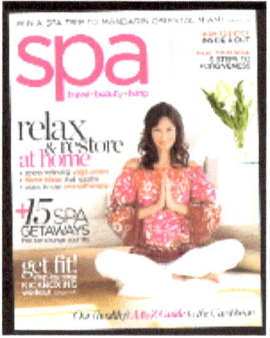

By: Anne-Marie Cook
Spa Magazine

Health Report—Creative Visualization
Want to drop pounds, quit smoking, or stress less? Then consider guided visualization. A technique used by psychologists since the late 1800s, it is now being offered at spas, too—such as Mezzanine Spa in New York City and The TreeHouse in Venice Beach, California – through a program called Creative Visualization and Relaxation (CVR). The brainchild of Dr. Patrick Porter, CVR utilizes flashing LEDs and sound pulses to guide you into a relaxed state bordering on sleep in which suggestions reach deeper than they can when the mind is alert. During each of the more than 300 CVR programs available, you are asked to visualize yourself in various scenarios to train your mind to react to old triggers with new behaviors. There's also a personal version that lets you take the power of positive thinking with you wherever you go.

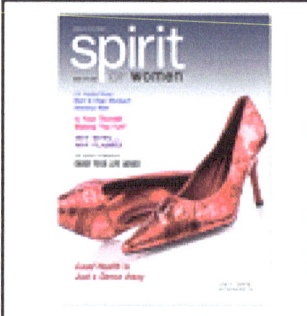

By: *Spirit of Women*
Spring 2008

Envision Yourself to Better Health
Guided imagery is similar to meditation, except that the focus of your thought is a physical part of the body you'd like to strengthen. The process of picturing a healthy heart or a svelte body can lower stress levels and help you "see" what it would feel like to be well.

High-tech Guided Imagery
You don't necessarily have to shell out big bucks for a personalized coach to reap the benefits of guided imagery . . . self-administered mental coaching programs can help you conquer bad habits or initiate good habits just by envisioning it—sitting back in your favorite easy chair, taking a deep breath, and completely relaxing every muscle in the body. A critical element . . . is light and sound technology to make your brain more receptive to the coaching. Just as the stimuli of music beats and flashing lights at a night club affect your brain . . . light and sound technology bring your brain frequency to a state called theta. The theta state is a meditative one that reportedly leads to higher levels of creativity, learning and inspiration.

The "Wellness Revolution" is Sweeping the Nation
Forward thinking hospitals that address patient demand for total wellness are now providing creative visualization and relaxation (CVR) mental coaching for their patients.

The Once-a-day Stress Relief Formula
"FOR ME AND ONLY ME"

By: *Lenny LaCour*
PULSE Magazine

Science proves that if you don't process your day-to-day experiences, they stay in your sub-conscious and keep you awake. Relaxation and exercise, yoga, music and the overall environment can help. It's getting back to the basics of the mind, body and spirit.

Dr. Patrick Porter explained that it's important to take a few minutes during the day to just unplug your phone and become consciously aware of your thoughts. If you slow down mentally, you become more aware of your unconscious thinking. Basically, we clog up our minds to the point where we can't focus on positive thoughts. Porter's theory is that our mind works in blocks of information. The conscious mind can only store several chunks at a time, and the rest of the thoughts remain in the subconscious waiting to be resolved. It's important to clear your mind to allow the wind to blow the thoughts through.

Dr. Porter's program is based on creative visualization and relaxation (CVR). Sessions result in stress release, clearer thinking, improved memory and enhanced creativity—a spiritual journey within yourself indeed.

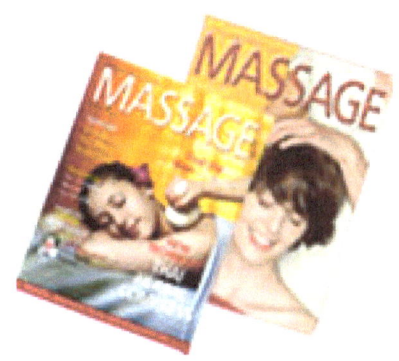

By: Chris Cunningham
Massage Magazine

The New Generation of Mind-Body Therapies—Biofeedback and Brain Training

Massage therapist Leslie White uses the biofeedin equipment and Dr. Patrick Porter's soothing voice to full advantage during her massage sessions. She said the combination of light, pulsating sound and "Dr. Porter's very pleasant voice softly saying, 'Now you will feel her hands massaging,'" really helps the clients "focus on themselves."

Meditation at the Mezzanine Spa

"After about 15 minutes, it was as though my mind and body were at one. It was similar to the feeling you get when you're almost asleep and then have a sort of "mini-dream" that brings you back to the waking world."

By: *Kelly Hushin*
BeautyNewsNYC.com

Researchers tested novice meditators on a button-pressing task requiring speed and concentration. Performance was greater after 40 minutes of meditation than after a 40-minute nap.

The Boston Globe
November 23, 2005

What the research has to say about Frequency Following Response...

Dr. Roger K. Cady, Dr. Norman Shealy in "Neurochemical Responses to Cranial Electrical Stimulation and Photo-Stimulation via Brain Wave Synchronization." Study performed by the Shealy Institute of Comprehensive Health Care, Springfield, Missouri, 1990, 11 pp.:

Eleven patients had peridural and blood analysis performed before and after the relaxation sessions using flash emitting goggles. An average increase of beta-endorphin levels of 25% and serotonin levels of 21% were registered. The beta-endorphin levels are comparative to those obtained by cranial electrical stimulation (CES). This indicates a potential decrease of depression related symptoms when using photic stimulation.

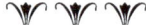

Dr. Norman Shealy, Dr. Richard Cox In `Pain Reduction and Relaxation with Brain Wave Synchronization (Photo-Stimulation). Study performed by the Forest Institute of Professional Psychology, Springfield, Missouri, 1990, 9pp.

Cerebral synchronization was obtained with photic stimulation devices and tested on more than 5,000 patients suffering from chronic pain and stress-symptoms during the `80s. A detailed study on 92 patients indicated that 88 obtained relaxation results higher than 60% after 30- minute sessions at 10 hz. Thirty patients had sessions in Theta (5 hz) and experienced relaxation states of 50-100% after five minutes as well as improved pain relief. Eight patients had blood tests before and after the sessions and showed improved beta-endorphin levels of 10-50%. All of these relaxation results are improved when combining the photic stimulation with relaxation audio tapes.

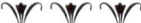

Dr. Thomas Budzynski in "Biofeedback and the Twilight States of Consciousness," in G.E. Schwartz and D. Shapiro eds., Consciousness and Self-Regulation, vol. 1, New York, Plenum 1976 and non-published studies at the Biofeedback Institute of Denver, 1980:

Using a first-generation prototype, Dr. Budzynski concluded that "these devices produce a distinct relaxation state. Programming the device between 3 and 7 hz, it takes about 10 to 15 minutes for the patients to enter--effortlessly-a state of hypnosis. They terminate the sessions relaxed and with a feeling of well-being." Also, "the device has a calming effect on nervous or anxious patients. In a majority of cases the patients feel relaxed and calm during a period of three to four days after the session. It happens that the subjects have a reminiscence of childhood experiences, particularly when in Theta. They related their experiences which we incorporated into our psychotherapeutic program."

Dr. Gene W. Brockopp, Review of Research on Multi-Modal Sensory Stimulation with Clinical Implications and Research Proposals (non-published,1984):

Dr. Brockopp analyzed audio-visual brain stimulation and in particular hemispheric synchronization during EEG monitoring. "By inducing hemispheric coherence the machine can contribute to improved intellectual functioning of the brain. Like children spending most of their time in Theta, the machine allows a reduction in learning time. With adults a return into Theta allows them to rediscover childhood experiences. The machine is like a `lost and found office' for the subconscious."

Dr. Brockopp's conclusion is that dissipative structures allow the mind-via audio-visual stimulation-to abandon certain present neurological structures in order to maintain a higher, more coherent and flexible state of consciousness, thus allowing for improved communication of neuro-entities.

Dr. Norman Thomas and David Siever, University of Alberta, Florida. Several publications, notably: The Effect of Repetitive Audio/Visual Stimulation in Skeletomotor and Vasomotor Activity, 1989:

"We stimulated one of two groups of 30 people with a brain- stimulation device to test relaxation levels, using 10 hz frequency while observing their muscular tension with an EMG and their index skin temperature. The second group had to relax without machines via traditional means of autosuggestion. Most of the people in the second group said they felt relaxed while demonstrating greater tension (EMG) and lower skin temperatures, both of which are stress and nervous tension indicators. The group using the machine obtained deep relaxation state going beyond the programmed 15 minutes. EMG curves confirmed relaxation of the cortex due to the frequency adoption response."

These findings were also verified by James Greene and Dr. E.J. Baukus of FOCUS Human Research Development in Bourdonnais, Illinois. The muscular tension curve of the trapezius muscle were indicative of deep muscular relaxation.

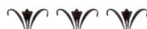

Dr. Robert Cosgrove, Jr. of the anesthesia department of Stanford University School of Medicine, Stanford, California.

Dr. Cosgrove proceeded in 1988 with multiple experiences with the same devices and concluded that states of deep relaxation are obtained with these machines. "We are very optimistic about the possibilities of calming our patients before and after surgery. By the way, we already treat chronic stress affected patients. Thus, our EEG analysis shows that optimal cerebral functioning can be obtained with regular use of such audio-visual apparatus. The machines could eventually slow the decreasing cerebral performance with the elderly. This type of machine could 'revolutionize neurology and medicine.'"

Dale S. Foster of Memphis State University, "EEG and Subjective Correlates of Alpha Frequency Binaural Beats Stimulation Combined with Alpha Biofeedback," 1988:

Mr. Foster's conclusions indicate that the combination of binaural sounds with audio-visual stimulation machines allow access into Alpha states of consciousness much faster than with traditional biofeedback techniques.

Elisabeth Philipos, Pepperdine University, California, and James McGaugh, University of California, Irvine, have tested the effects of Theta frequencies on learning.

During their study a group of 20 students learned 1,800 words of Bulgarian in 120 hours while using Theta stimulation programs. In about 1/3 of normal time they spoke and wrote the new language.

D.J. Anderson, B.Sc., M.B., "The Treatment of Migraine with Variable Frequency Photo-Stimulation," in Headache, March 1989, pp 154-155:
D.J. Anderson used photo-stimulating goggles with variable frequency using red LEDs in order to stimulate the optic nerve, through closed eyes, right and left with frequencies between 0.5 and 50 hz. The study included seven patients who suffered a total of more than 50 migraines during the observation period. Forty-nine of these migraines were relieved (either by reducing the average duration or by increasing the frequency interval in between migraine crisis) and 36 other migraines could be stopped while using the goggles.

Dr. Glen D. Solomon, "Slow Wave Photic Stimulation in the Treatment of Headache-A Preliminary Report," in Headache, November 1985, pp 444-447:
Dr. Solomon works for the Department of Internal Medicine at the U.S. Air Force Medical Center in Scott, Illinois, where 24 patients with chronic headaches and migraines were treated with photic stimulation apparatus at 5-8 hz frequency. Fourteen of 15 patients with sustained headaches and 5 of 6 patients with chronic headaches noticed complete relief after the treatment. Four patients treated with the same photo- stimulation apparatus showed no reaction.

Bruce Harrah-Confort, Ph.D., Indiana University, "Alpha and Theta Response to the MindsEye Plus," 1990:
The study included 15 persons between the ages of 24 and 38 years old who were asked to relax via auto-suggestion with headphones dispensing a synthetic sound (100 cycles at 60 hz) and then to use the audio-visual stimulator MindsEye PlusTM. EEG graphic analysis showed that the first relaxation method did not alter the EEG-trace significantly vs. normal. MindsEye Plus users had, however, strongly improved Alpha and Theta tracings and experienced profound relaxation. There were also signs that would validate hemispheric synchronization during the experience.

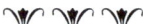

Joseph Glickson, Department of Psychology, Tel Aviv University, "Photic Driving and Altered States of Consciousness: An Exploratory Study," in Imagination, Cognition and Personality, vol. 6(2), 1986-87, pp 167-182:
Four persons were exposed to photic stimulation in the 18, 10 and 6 hz ranges. A frequency response was established by two subjects during the initial session according to EEG measurements. These persons had an altered state of consciousness, and reported their visual and auditive experiences. The two other subjects had similar experiences during follow-on sessions. The study concludes that photic entrainment provokes altered states of consciousness according to the applied frequencies.

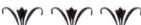

Paul Williams and Michael West, Department of Psychological Medicine, University Hospital of Wales and University of Wales Institute of Science and Technology, Cardiff, Wales, "EEG Responses to Photic Stimulation in Persons Experienced in Meditation," in Electroencephalography and Clinical Neurophysiology, 1975, 39, pp 519-522:
Williams and West tested photic entrainment on two test groups of 10 people. The test group produced significantly more Alpha waves and smaller Alpha blocking compared to the control group familiar with traditional meditation techniques. Alpha induction was realized faster and more frequently within the test vs. the control group.

Tsuyoshi Inouye, Noboru Sumitsuji and Kazuo Matsumoto, Department of Neuropsychiatry, Osaka University Medical School, Japan, "EEG Changes Induced by Light Stimuli Modulated with the Subject's Alpha Rhythm," in Electroencephalography and Clinical Neurophysiology, 1980, 49, pp 135-142:
Seven of nine persons undergoing the test obtained occipital Alpha of both hemispheres and concurrently coherence and phase between right and left occipital EEG. These results tend to confirm a hemispheric synchronization tendency by subjects using photic stimulation in the 10 hz (Alpha frequency) range.

Ronald Lesser, Hans Luders, G. Klem and Dudley Dinner, Department of Neurology, Cleveland Clinic Foundation, "Visual Potentials Evoked by Light- Emitting Diodes Mounted in Goggles," in Cleveland Clinic Quarterly, vol. 52, No. 2, Summer 1985, pp. 223-228:
A comparison of stimulation by strobiscopic lights and LED diodes shows that both methods have similar effects. LED stimulation may be preferable in intensive care units or during surgery because the type of stimulus is less disturbing.

Richard E. Townsend, Ph.D. of Neuropsychiatric Research, U.S. Naval Hospital in San Diego, "A Device for Generation and Presentation of Modulated Light Stimuli," in Electroencephalography and Clinical Neurophysiology, 1973, 34, pp 97-99:
The author describes a system allowing generation and presentation of modulated light stimuli with variable frequencies and wave forms. He concludes the possibilities of stimulation and positive responses during sleep-preparation and insomnia troubles.

Dr. William Harris, Director of the Penwell Foundation, USA in 1990:
Preliminary studies with audio-visual brain stimulators used by patients with AIDS indicate that "the devices are extremely efficient in terms of providing mental clarity, improved sleeping patterns (for sleep preparation and sleep duration) allowing for better physical disintoxication by the liver. The apparatus also stimulates immunology functions through states of deep relaxation."

Dr. Olivier Carreau, Saint-Louis Hospital in Paris, on "Efficiency of the MindsEye Plus audio-visual stimulator in treatment of the psoriasis during puvatherapy," study completed in January 1991.
Dr. Carreau analyzed 20 patients over a period of five months. Patients were treated one per week alternately via UVA and audio-visual stimulation (30-minute sessions) for psychosomatic skin disorders. All patients experienced deep relaxation during the sessions and had a feeling of well-being during the entire day. Five patients claimed that this feeling lasted for the following 2-3 days. Patients with combined therapy did better than with puvatherapy alone.

Books Featuring Self-Mastery Technology

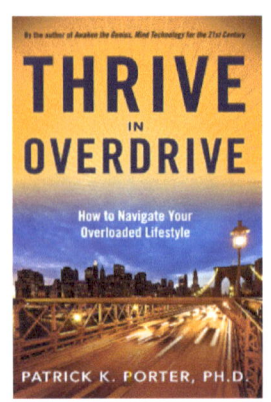

Thrive in Overdrive
How to Navigate Your Overloaded Lifestyle
Patrick K. Porter, Ph.D.

In today's high-tech, fast-paced world, no one is immune to stress. Why? Because our lives are too overloaded. Thrive in Overdrive shows you how to rid yourself of the happiness-robbing condition called stress and enjoy a balanced life, but without giving up your overdrive lifestyle that makes sure you stay ahead of the game. The book, written by recognized how-to self-help expert, Dr. Patrick Porter, is based on methods that have been time-tested by over a million clients worldwide. He uses true stories, anecdotes, and deceivingly simple creative visualization exercises to demonstrate that, yes, you can have it all.

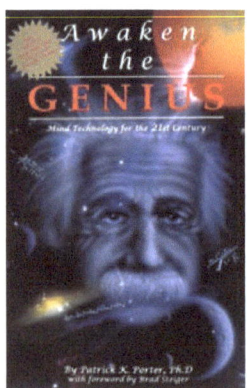

Awaken the GeniusMind Technology for the 21st Century
Patrick K. Porter, Ph.D.

You'll discover how to maintain a Genuine positive attitude...how to unleash your personal passion and Enthusiasm (including stories and fun-to-do exercises)...how to develop Non-stop enrgy and center that energy on reaching your goals...how to activate your unlimited imagination and creativity...how to enjoy and unending drive to succeed...and...how to experience every day what geniuses throughout history have enjoyed-spontaneous intuitive breakthroughs.

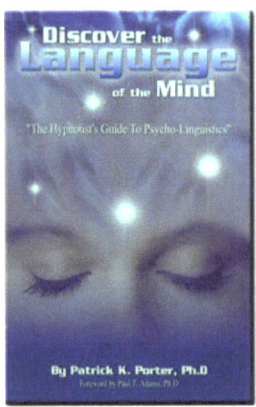

Discover the Language of the Mind
Patrick K. Porter, Ph.D.

Discover the Language of the Mind, the Hypnotist's Guide to Psycho-Linguistics was previously published as Psycho-Linguistics, The Language of the Mind. This fully revised edition includes updates on dozens of new developments in the hypnosis field, full transcripts for each of the eleven processes, which includes two never-before published techniques as developed and tested by Dr. Patrick Porter. Psycho-Linguistics is a practical guide to the combined theories of hypnosis, Neuro-Linguistic Programming, Creative Visualization and Accelerated Learning - a perfect 'mind guide' for experienced hypnotists and psychotherapists or for anyone seeking a quick, easy, step-by-step method for self-improvement and enhanced communication.

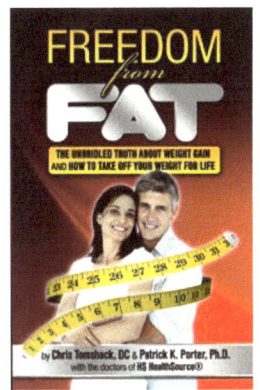

Freedom From Fat
The Unbridled Truth about Weight Gain and How to Take off Your Weight for Life
Patrick K Porter, Ph.D.

Chris Tomshack, DC

And the Doctors at HealthSource® Chiropractctic

This is not another diet book! Rather, it's your chance to finally understand why you're gaining weight and how to reverse the cycle. By following the advice of these doctors, you can achieve safe, healthy and lasting weight loss success. If you're looking for a real world, step-by-step plan for taking off your weight and keeping it off, brought to you by doctors who are helping patients succeed even when all else has failed, this book is your answer.

Within these pages you will discover:
- *Why fad diets, gimmicks and complicated diet plans are doomed from the start*
- *The underlying condition that makes it nearly impossible for some people to lose weight, and how to fix it*
- *A system that addresses every part of the weight puzzle-diet, mental attitude, habits*
- *How to change the core causes of cravings, conditioned overeating, and weight gain so you can keep your weight off for life*

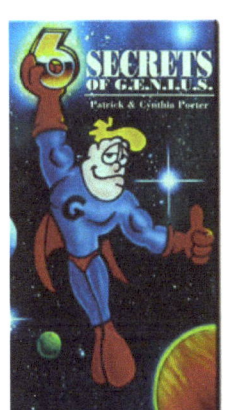

Six Secrets of G. E. N. I. U. S.
Patrick K. Porter, Ph.D.

Cynthia J. Porter, Ph.D.

Discover what inventors, artists and other great minds have known for centuries-the secrets of sparking their own creativity and super-charging their motivation. Learn simple strategies to rid yourself of negative thinking...to awaken your positive attitude in every situation...and to think your way through complex or confusing challenges. Discover what inventors, artists and other great minds have known for centuries-the secrets of sparking their own creativity and super-charging their motivation. Learn simple strategies to rid yourself of negative thinking...to awaken your positive attitude in every situation...and to think your way through complex or confusing challenges.

Weight Loss For Life in 10 Easy Steps
Todd Singelton, DC
Patrick K. Porter, Ph.D

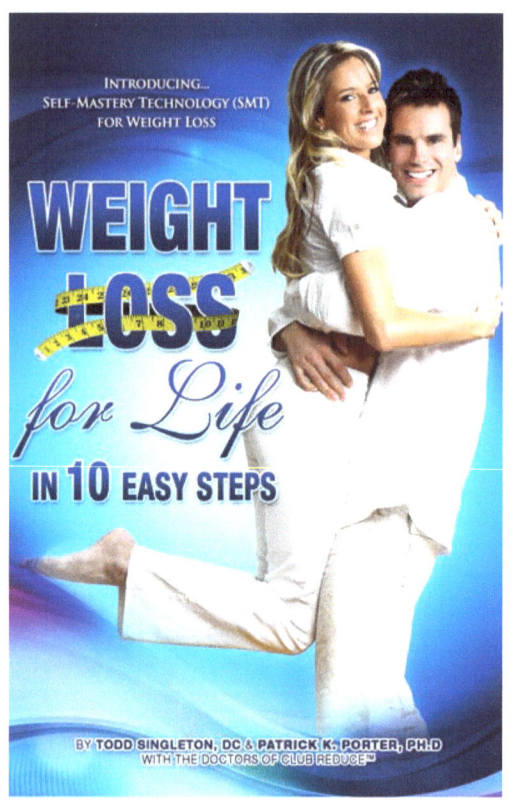

If you could lose weight on your own, you wouldn't be holding this book in your hands right now. The experts all tell you to eat fewer calories and exercise more. If only it were that easy! The truth is, most people and most so-called experts have no idea what triggers the body to gain or lose weight. Few people recognize the clues (symptoms) that are your body's warning signals that your food choices aren't working. Add the fact that almost no one understands the relationship between stress and weight, and it's no wonder we have a nation of chronic dieters who stay overweight, unhealthy and unhappy no matter how hard they try. Well, today is your day...because you have in your hands the definitive guidebook for weight loss success that lasts. Within these pages we'll teach you everything you need to know to lose weight and keep it off for life, and it couldn't be simpler when all you have to do is follow ten easy steps! Together, we'll finally make your dream a reality so you can...

- *Stop starving*
- *Be rid of cravings*
- *End emotional eating*
- *Turn off fat storage hormones*
- *Supercharge fat burning hormones*
- *Suppress your appetite naturally*
- *Clear up digestive problems*
- *Reverse the stress/weight effect*
- *Do away with habitual overeating*
- *Achieve radiant good health from the inside out!.*

Welcome to The Gift of Love Project

The Gift of Love is a poetic writing that has its own beauty … and upon further examination, it may lead one to a contemplative process, creating balance and harmony in one's everyday life. Over time, this process can also create subtle positive change in the recipient of **The Gift**.

My guidance leads me to distribute this writing to one billion people within the next two years. Hopefully, many people will be led to practice the contemplative process. If **The Gift of Love** resonates with you, please share it with others. As we gather and hold the **power of love** in our consciousness, we will dramatically reduce the level of anger, fear, and hatred on our planet today. -- Jerry DeShazo

The Gift of Love

I Agree Today
To Be The Gift of Love.

I Agree to Feel Deeply
Love for Others
Independent of Anything
They Are Expressing,
Saying, Doing, or Being.

I Agree to Allow Love
As I Know It
To Embrace My Whole Body
And Then to Just Send It
To Them Silently and Secretly.

I Agree to Feel it, Accept it, Breathe It
Into Every Cell of My Body on Each In-Breath
And On Each Out-Breath
Exhale Any Feeling Unlike Love.

I Will Repeat This Breathing Process Multiple Times
Until I Feel it Fully and Completely
Then Consciously Amplify In Me
The Feeling of Love and Project It to Others
As The Gift of Love.

This is My Secret Agreement –
No One Else Is To Know it.

This page may be reproduced in totality
for any peaceful purpose without financial gain.
All rights reserved, Jerome DeShazo, D.D., M.B.A.,M.C.C.

For more about The Gift of Love Project and to view the videos, please visit www.TheGiftofLove.com. You will also be given access to a special 9-minute Creative Visualization that will align you with the **Power of Love** and supercharge your day. Together we will change the world one person at a time.

http://www.thegiftoflove.com/

www.ingramcontent.com/pod-product-compliance
Lightning Source LLC
Chambersburg PA
CBHW041529220426
43671CB00002B/31